The Reach for the Ring

The Reach for the Ring

my 42 year love affair with the iron

jon m ketcham

The Reach for the Ring - my 42 year love affair with the iron
by jon

© 2020 by **Jon M. Ketcham**. All rights reserved.

ABIYD Publishing Company
www.ABIYD.com

Illustrations by Jon D. Ketcham

ISBN: 978-0-9905511-5-7 paperback
Library of Congress Control Number: 2020914651

10 9 8 7 6 5 4 3 2 1

Bodybuilding & Weight Training / Inspiration & Personal Growth

First Edition Printed in Saegertown, PA, United States.

Additional Disclaimer

The information and strategies provided by **The Reach for the Ring** are intended to educate, inform, empower, amuse and inspire you on your personal journey towards excellence in bodybuilding & weight training. They are based upon the author's personal experience, over a 42-year period, with what worked best for him alone. It is clearly not intended to replace a one-on-one relationship with a personal trainer, nor a licensed health care professional and it is definitely not offered up as a substitute for proper medical or chiropractic advice, diagnosis or treatment. Proper diagnosis and advice relative to treatment of any existing health conditions cannot be made through a book and is well beyond the scope of any information offered. The intent of the author is solely to offer information of a general nature to assist you on your quest for physical perfection. The author will not accept any liability, perceived or otherwise, for the improper application of any principles taught through this text. In the event you, the reader, choose to use or apply any of the strategies in this book for yourself, which is your constitutional right, the publisher and the author assume no responsibility for your actions.

The Reach for the Ring

Dedication

Steve Musiek was a pioneer in the truest sense of the word. He had a championship-level physique decades before it became commonplace. There were no commercial gyms when he developed his work of art, only the local Y.M.C.A. I can remember Steve telling me about how, once he brought a weight set of his own in for the high school football team that he coached to train with, only to have the school board members promptly make him take the weights away, reprimanding him, "you'll ruin those kids!"

It is solely due to the efforts of people like Steve Musiek and Jack LaLanne that such incidents are unfathomable today. High schools today have better training facilities than anything Steve could have imagined training on for himself. He shared his passion for bodybuilding with anyone willing to listen. Steve was the perpetual spokesperson for the benefits of lifelong training and living the bodybuilding lifestyle. He was one of my earliest idols in bodybuilding and certainly the first one I knew personally with such a magnificent physique. Over the years, he became a mentor, good friend and, at times, father figure to me as well. A year or so before he passed, Steve told me, completely out of the blue, that he would have been proud to have me as a son.

I love and miss you Steve. This book is for you.

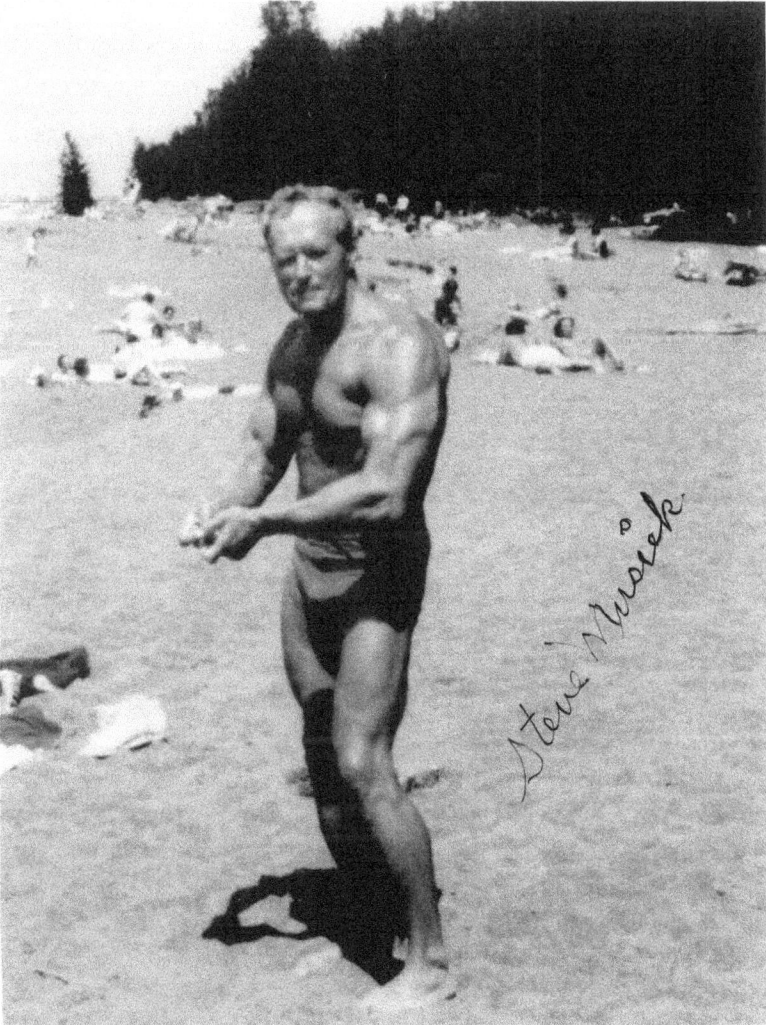

Steve at 70 years old

The Reach for the Ring

Table of Contents

Disclaimers   *iv,v*

Dedication   *vii*

Table of Contents   *xi*

Preface   *xiii*

Chapter 1 The Basics   1

Chapter 2 Busted... Myths & Folklore   13

Chapter 3 Much Ado About Nothing   19

Chapter 4 Finding True Love   23

Chapter 5 Body Drag Curls   29

Chapter 6 Starting Over   33

Chapter 7 Rehab & Prehab   39

Chapter 8 Spotting Fails   49

Chapter 9 Character Assessment   57

Chapter 10 Benefits of a Home Gym   63

Chapter 11 Rotations & Routines   67

Chapter 12 Sculpting David   135

Chapter 13 Mousetraps   147

About the Author   *153*

Bodybuilding Resume   *157*

Connecting with the Author   *161*

Other Books by jon m ketcham   *163*

Appendix A - Patent Documents   *165*

Appendix B - CAD Drawings   *175*

Appendix C - KC Row Bench Prototype *187*

Preface

During the late 1800s and continuing into the early-to-mid 1900s, carousel riders at amusement parks, riding on the outside row of horses, were provided with the challenge of reaching for a ring, released at random by a dispenser, as the carousel turned. Most of the rings were iron, but one or two per ride were brass. Acquiring the brass ring entitled the recipient to a prize, usually a free ride, as well as bragging rights to their peers. Over the years, reaching for the brass ring has become synonymous with striving for the highest prize and living a life of excellence. Such is the intent in titling this book, The Reach for the Ring, as it represents my 42-year involvement with the iron game.

Chapter 1

The Basics

Some people are born to lift heavy weights,
some are born to juggle golden balls.
Max Beerbohm

This is not your basic "how to" guide to exercising. The Reach for the Ring assumes a fundamental understanding of weight training, bodybuilding, powerlifting, etc. I will not be covering basic terminology like sets and reps nor will I be covering most exercises and their proper performance. There are a plethora of books and internet websites that already cover those topics in far greater detail and much more eloquently than I could ever hope to. What The Reach for the Ring has to offer that the others do not is my 42 years of experience in the realms of bodybuilding and weight training, the nuances and tidbits that can take your training to the next level, along with numerous stories and anecdotes that I have accumulated over the years that can make your training more meaningful and productive. I will also attempt to dispel a number of the bullshit myths that continue to proliferate.

First and foremost, it is imperative that you always have a plan! Know your why behind every rep, of every set, of every exercise, of every workout that you perform. What are your short and long-term goals? For instance, when I train my back, I always include one exercise for width, one exercise for thickness and, as my training cycle progresses, I may add in a shaping or finishing movement. Speaking of training cycles, are you at the beginning, middle or end of a given training cycle? In the early stages of a new workout program, you want to start slowly and not push yourself too hard. Most of the strength gains, in the first few weeks of a new program, are primarily due to awakening new neurologic pathways and recruiting more muscle fibers than due to any actual muscular improvements. As you progress through a training cycle, you can ramp up the intensity with which you push yourself. After you reach a peak in any given training cycle, you should plan in a period of added rest and recovery. For myself, I typically factor in a week off after every 3-6 months of training, depending upon the body part. As for waiting until you get to the gym and just doing whatever exercise hits your fancy, what they call instinctive training, or worse, just performing every exercise you can think of, I'm personally not a big fan of either one of these approaches.

Next, how will you measure your progress? I am a huge fan of always documenting your workouts in a workout log or journal. The benefits of keeping a workout journal are many. Workout-to-workout, you don't have to rely on memory as to how many reps and sets, and with how much weight, you performed last time. For example, if I see that last week I used 185 pounds on Incline Presses for 15 reps on my final set, I now have a visual record, something to strive against this time. I can now choose to attempt to match what I did last time, increase my reps, increase the weight and decrease the reps, increase the weight and match the reps, or even just move through my chest routine in a shorter amount of time. Don't underestimate the value of this practice. Over time, keeping records such as this allows you to spot trends, keep records of new max weights used, track the results of new training programs and refer back to in times of starting over. I have kept records of every one of my workouts since 1980.

But training itself is only one part of the equation. Equal consideration must be given to your post-workout recovery. The key to sustained growth, over time, is not how much training you can do, in terms of volume, frequency and/or intensity; rather, it's how much training you can recover from. This varies widely from one individual to another. Developing a full and proper understanding of this one concept will make or break your training results. In fact, *this is the most important concept I will share in this entire book. It's that important!* Think of your recovery from training as existing along a continuum. Lots of things exert influence over whether you maximally recover from your workout session or not, only some of which are under your control.

In the ideal scenario, you train hard and then you maximally recover session after session after session, getting bigger and stronger along the way. But then there are outside stressors like work, poor eating habits and insufficient sleep. And don't forget about the role genetics play in recovery ability. In the less than ideal scenario, you end up overtraining, which can actually cause muscle loss instead of muscle gain. Left unchecked, this can lead to illness and/or injury and, in extreme cases, irreversible damage to your health and even death. However, for most trainees, it just means no growth. *[See RM Meter Diagram at end of chapter]*.

There's a saying, common among people who train, that there's no such thing as overtraining, only under-eating and under-sleeping. That's really not the case though. I personally experimented, off and on for about one year, with low dosages of steroids in the mid-to-late '80s. It was a phenomenal learning experience for me. For the first time in over 6 years of training, I experienced what it actually felt like to maximally recover from a workout. I was able to train as intensely as I chose to, for as long as I chose to, and still maximally recover. I also got to see, first hand, how others responded while using steroids. I met a man who had gained over 100 pounds in only 6 years. I also witnessed the high injury rates that plagued those who used steroids. Muscle growth and strength tend to increase at a faster rate than tendon and ligament strength; subsequently, pec tears and bicep tears were commonplace. I only experimented with steroids for about one year, but it was long enough to radically alter the way I trained for the rest of my life. High intensity techniques like forced reps and negatives were now out for me; I had not been able to recover from them in the past and now it was clear that chemical assistance was the only way I would be able to. Furthermore, I learned to always end each set, and workout, on a positive note. I learned to complete the last rep that I could by myself and then be done. As Bill Pearl advocates, I learned to always leave a little gas in the gas tank at the end of every workout so that I left the gym feeling invigorated rather than near death every time.

There are a lot of different training methodologies out there and they all have some merit. When choosing which one to follow, it's important to always evaluate each based upon a cost/benefit analysis. Heavy Duty training, for example, as advocated by Mike Mentzer and Dorian Yates, allows you to max out your genetic potential faster than other methods but it also carries a much higher injury risk than more traditional training methods, often career-ending injuries. High Intensity

Interval Training (HIIT) is another very popular methodology that is very efficient for weight loss. It tends to be more muscle sparing than lower intensity cardio methods, but it also creates a very high systemic load, increasing the chances of overtraining. I have trained using both methods at various times in my career but I have not been able to tolerate either one for any length of time without becoming very ill as a result.

This is my training philosophy in a nutshell: *the human body is designed to be in motion.* I have never taken an extended break from training that I did not regret later; injuries become more entrenched and functionality decreases over time the longer you go without training, particularly as you get older. Even after my near fatal burst appendix episode back in 2001, I was up and moving again, within injury dictated boundaries, very quickly.

The important thing is that you find a training methodology that will allow you train consistently, for the long term, without overtraining. The muscle magazines that were popular when I was coming up the ranks in bodybuilding in the 1980s and 1990s often promoted 20 sets per body part, training 6 days per week and training each body part 2-3 times per week. Without the aid of steroids, which enable such high intensity training to be anabolic instead of catabolic, I never would have been able to follow such a program. Instead, training naturally, I found that I did best with no more than 8-10 sets for large body parts like legs and back, no more than 5-6 sets for smaller body parts like arms, training only 4-5 days per week and only training each body part once every 5-7 days. For most body parts, I perform only 2 exercises: 1 compound movement for size and 1 isolation movement for shape. There are a couple of exceptions here: back, where I perform 2 size movements, 1 for width and 1 for thickness, along with 1 isolation movement for shape, is one such exception. Forearms and abs are the other exceptions where, for forearms I typically perform 1 movement for flexors and 1 movement for extensors, and for abs, I perform 1 exercise for lower abs and 1 exercise for upper abs. You have to find the balance that works best for you.

The Reach for the Ring

RM Meter

A VU meter, or volume unit meter, is an analog device used to measure the signal levels in audio equipment. It consists of a needle that moves in response to the volume of input. If the input is too high, it jumps into the red zone. Prior to the digital age, these were common in all stereo equipment. My stereo, back in the late 1970s had them in both the cassette deck and the receiver. Imagine if you could have an RM meter, a recovery meter, that worked along the same principle and could measure your level of recovery following each workout. The measurement needle would have, as its starting point, the beginning of your workout. To the left of the starting point would be no recovery (overtraining), negative recovery (muscle loss, illness/injury) and finally severe negative recovery (permanent damage and/or death; e.g. rhabdomyolysis). To the right of the starting point would be good recovery and maximal recovery. Since maximal recovery following each workout is the ultimate goal, it could be represented as the brass ring, the highest prize and living a life of excellence. Numerous variables must be taken into consideration for how they will influence the movement of the needle.

The Reach for the Ring

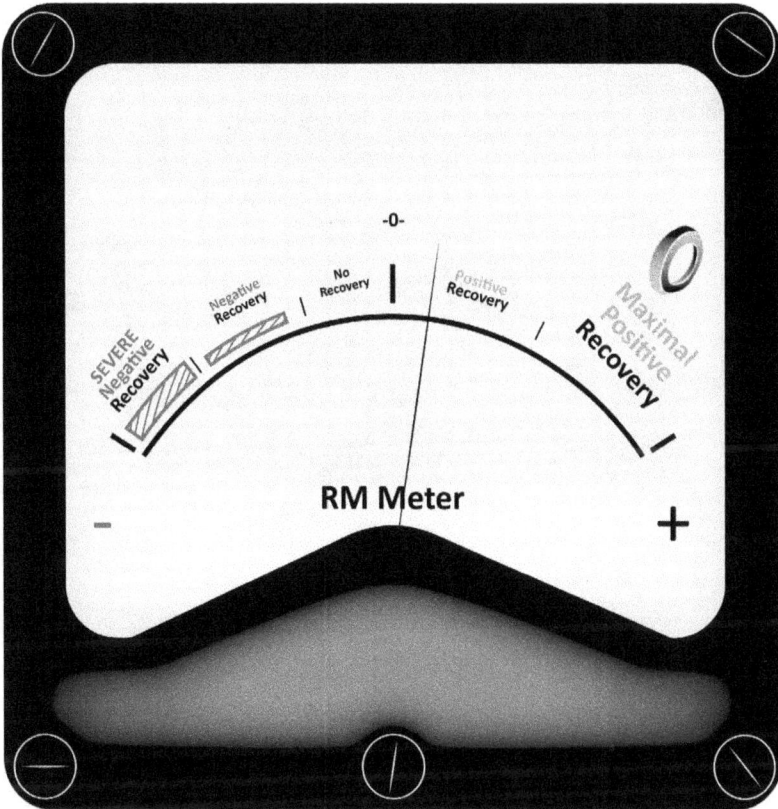

To the left:
- poor nutrition & inadequate rest
- bad habits (e.g. smoking, drinking)
- insufficient training history
- exceeding personal recovery ability

To the right:
- good nutrition & adequate rest
- training within personal recovery ability
- steroids

The Reach for the Ring

Chapter 2

Busted... Myths & Folklore

If the truth were self-evident,
eloquence would be unnecessary.
Cicero

When I began my journey 42 years ago, there was no internet. Everything I learned about bodybuilding and weight training came from reading muscle magazines and any books I could lay my hands on, personal experimentation and listening to the experiences of others. Much of what I read and listened to was based more upon myths and folklore than actual reality. With the advent of the internet and literally unlimited amounts of information at our fingertips, sadly, very little has changed. The more things change, the more they stay the same actually. I will do my best to dispel some of the more outrageous myths and folklore with this chapter.

You have to keep getting stronger to get bigger.

No, you don't! Size and strength are really not directly correlated. I can remember, before the '93 Can/Am Bodybuilding Championship, being told about a fellow competitor who I would be facing in my weight class. Several guys at the gym I was training at knew him and warned me in advance that he had a 500-pound squat. I was just barely able to squat 250 pounds at the time. And yet, I had no difficulty beating him in competition. That's not a commentary on the other man's physique; he was very well developed too. It's just to point out that how much he could squat didn't matter that day. My good friend, Carl Devries, an accomplished bodybuilder with a pro-level physique of his own, taught me that, for bodybuilding, it's not how much you can lift, it's how much you look like you can lift. Learning how to make the mind/muscle link is the key.

If you miss a workout you will shrink.

Early in my lifting career, I used to think this. In fact, the more consistent my workouts became, the more I feared shrinking if I ever missed a workout. Not only was this irrational, but it crossed the line into addiction. How bad was it? I once tried to convince a gym owner to let me train in the dark during an ice storm. I also let it spoil a camping trip because I couldn't be too far from the gym. And I quit my first job after college rather than have to work the pending 3 months of mandatory overtime because I didn't want to miss a workout. The truth is that you don't shrink after missing only a day, or even a week, of training. Even if you do have a prolonged amount of time off, thanks to muscle memory, you can always get back what you lost if you're willing to put in the time and effort.

Nowadays, I plan time off in my rotations, typically 1 week after every 3-6 months of training; but even after prolonged periods of time off due to illness, injury, chiropractic school, etc., I can honestly say that it has always come back as long as I don't rush it and create new injuries in the process.

Supine triceps extensions (skull krushers) are NOT a size move for triceps.

I actually stopped doing these for a period of time after reading this, despite the fact that my prior training history said otherwise. Numerous sources I encountered said that, for triceps, close grip bench presses are the best size move whereas skull krushers are an isolation move and, therefore not a size move. Never mind the fact that close grip bench presses irritated my shoulders and did next to nothing for my triceps. Never mind the fact that most of my triceps mass, up to that point, had come from skull krushers, directly, and Incline presses, indirectly.

I eventually returned to doing skull krushers and my gains returned as well. The point is that you have to listen to your own body and act accordingly. I always lower the bar behind my head rather than to my forehead as that's what feels most natural to me.

You have to be training your legs, squats specifically, and subsequently gaining weight/size everywhere if you want your arms to grow.

I'm not even sure where to begin with this one, such utter nonsense. There is a segment of people in bodybuilding and weight training who literally worship at the altar of squatting, considering it the be-all and end-all of everything training related. The best example I can give here, and I have many, is a man I used to train with nearly 30 years ago named Chris. Chris had spectacular arm development; hell, his entire upper body was spectacular: wide, thick lats; full, well-developed pecs; broad, capped shoulders; thick, powerful triceps; huge, peaked biceps and a tiny waist that he could display with one of the best vacuum poses I have ever seen. Did I mention that Chris is a paraplegic? End of story.

Conventional wisdom says that, for growth, quads respond best to heavy weight, low reps whereas calves respond best to low weight, high reps.

Early in my weight training career, I squatted 365 pounds for sets of 6 reps. My legs were strong AND skinny! Later in my career, due to a series of lower back injuries, I was forced to use much lighter weight for higher reps. That is when, at long last, my quads actually began to grow. In fact, my quads grew their most in 1993 when I was training for the '93 Can/Am and I squatted considerably less weight. You can follow that particular series of workouts in Chapter 11, Rotations & Routines. As for calves, I have written the entire next chapter dispelling this one myth.

Leg presses are a poor substitute for squats.

I loved squatting when I was able to do so, but squatting never liked me and, in retrospect, probably was not an appropriate exercise choice for my particular structure; that's the consensus from multiple disc herniations anyway. In addition to experiencing my maximum quad growth while squatting lighter and for higher reps, the other factor that was in play was the fact that I began doing a lot of leg presses around the same time. All of the quad growth I ultimately accomplished I attribute to the lighter weight, higher reps that I performed on both squats and leg presses. If I would have switched over completely to leg presses 25 years ago, I might have avoided the disc injuries.

The bottom line is this: you have to learn, through your own trial and error, what doesn't work, what does work and what works best for you. Everyone is different. And, what works best for you today might not work as well, or at all, for you tomorrow. Keep an open mind and learn to listen to your individual body, always training within your own individual recovery ability.

Chapter 3

Much Ado About Nothing

Be what you are. This is the first step
toward becoming better than you are.
Julius Charles Hare

When I first began working out with weights, on
Christmas Day 1978, gyms were relatively rare
around where I lived. Weight training had yet to gain
mainstream acceptance. In fact, I first started lifting
weights against the recommendation of my boxing
coach, who assured me that it would make me slow
and inflexible. A chance encounter with one of the
older boxers in our boxing club changed the entire
trajectory my life would take from that point forward.
Gary was known as a knockout puncher, having won
most of his bouts in that manner. But, what stood out
most to me, as a starry-eyed 13 year old, was the
massive size of his chest and arms. I asked him one
day how he got his chest and arms so big. "Lifting
weights," he replied. "But, Lou told us not to lift
weights." "So, don't tell Lou!" was his response. And
so my journey turned.

The internet was still 20 long years away from
existence, so I was relegated to learning everything I
could about weight training through my own trial and

error methods. My first weight set was a 110 pound plastic Ultra-K-tron set from K-mart, a gift from my parents. Money was tight that year, more so than usual, and my parents asked each of us kids what we most wanted if we could only have one item from our Christmas list; a set of weights was mine, something my parents had originally not planned on getting for me because they didn't take me seriously when I had first asked and they didn't want a bunch of old weights sitting around collecting dust. Included with the weight set was a small booklet of barbell and dumbell exercises, by Bruce Randall, Mr. Universe, that provided instruction on beginner, intermediate and advanced exercises.

One of the exercises in the beginner course proved to be particularly challenging to me: toe raises. According to the booklet, or at least according to how I understood it at the time, the process was as follows: *standing with feet shoulder width apart, take a wide grip on the barbell that is on the floor and clean it from floor to chest. Press the weight overhead and then slowly lower the weight behind your head, resting it across your shoulders. Next, raise up on your toes and hold for a 2 count before returning to the floor. Repeat for 10 reps.*

So, again, having no other real basis for comparison, I did EXACTLY as it had instructed: cleaning the weight from floor to chest, pressing it overhead, slowly lowering it behind my neck, raising up on my toes for a 2 count and then pressing the weight from behind my head to overhead, lowering it back down in front and *returning the barbell back to the floor* after each and every rep! That's right, every set of 10 reps of toe raises that I did included 20 reps of shoulder presses and 10 reps of cleans; and that's after having already done a standing military press exercise earlier in the workout. In my defense, the course specifically instructed, *"Do not clean the weight with each repetition."* for the military presses. No such instruction accompanied the toe raises. My shoulders burned and grew like crazy from this particular workout, my calves not so much.

Calves would prove to be an exceptionally difficult muscle group for me to see any progress in whatsoever for many, many years. Even in the early 1990s, when I was competing successfully in natural bodybuilding contests, I was told by the judges, "You really need to bring your calves up," to which I would jokingly reply, "This is up!" Then, one day, I read an article in a muscle magazine where Arnold Schwarzenegger claimed to have learned how to develop his lagging calves after visiting Reg Park in South Africa. According to the article, Reg Park, also a Mr. Universe winner, told Arnold that, due to their fiber type and density, calves grow best with very heavy weights and relatively low reps, which was counter to the prevailing conventional wisdom of the day. Park argued that, for a 200 pound man, every step he takes hits that single calf with a 200 pound load, hence, anything less than 400 pounds on a standing calf raise would barely be noticed by his calves. And, according to this article, Arnold implemented Reg Park's advice and his calves grew to legendary proportions.

It made perfect sense to me so, in 2000, I started training my calves very heavy too, starting with 405 pounds and eventually working my way up to 585 pounds for sets of 6-8 reps. And, my calves improved significantly. They didn't grow to become legendary. They didn't even grow to equal my upper arm and neck girth, like most symmetry and proportion gurus recommend, but they grew significantly for me nonetheless.

One caveat regarding the story about Arnold and Reg Park: in recent years, there've been rumors floating around about calf implants. We may never know the truth about that one way or another. And, maybe it was just because it was such a radical shift in the way I had trained my calves previously, but using weight equal to or greater than double my bodyweight on standing calf raises for lower reps made all the difference in the world for my calf development.

Chapter 4

Finding True Love

Love is in the eye of the beholder.
Unknown

Who can say how it happens, or when or why? You finally find "the one." She makes your palms sweat in anticipation. She just "feels right." She builds you up like no other. You think about her all of the time and, when you're apart, you ache for her. I remember when I first found her. Who could have guessed, I knew her before, but I hadn't recognized her... until... It was so obvious, she was right there in front of me. But I didn't see it until...

I was competing in my very first bodybuilding competition, the '87 Oil City Y.M.C.A. Bodybuilding Championship. I.F.B.B. Professional David Hawk, a bodybuilder from Pittsburgh, was the guest poser. He also gave a training seminar during the intermission between the morning prejudging and the evening finals. I remember it like it was yesterday. David explained how he never did flat bench presses; said that, with his wide shoulders, bench pressing caused him more shoulder irritation than anything else. Instead, he relied upon inclines mostly, and declines, to develop his massive chest.

23

Bench presses had always irritated my wide shoulders too. If David Hawk didn't need to do bench presses, neither did I. Why hadn't I thought of this before? Inclines and declines it was then! I almost felt naughty, doing inclines exclusively, instead of flat bench presses. They were infinitely more comfortable, definitely more suited to my body structure, no shoulder discomfort whatsoever. I felt strong as a Mack truck doing them. And, let's face it, who couldn't use more upper chest development? Inclines became my "main squeeze" and have remained so for the ensuing 33 years.

The stories I could tell. I can remember one time, I was living in Canandaigua, NY, and I had just gotten to the gym, had the incline bench set up and everything, when the lights went out. The Fitness Factory, where I trained, was located in the basement under one of the buildings on the main street, accessible only through the back alley, and had no windows at all. Power outages meant absolutely no way to see inside whatsoever; there were no cell phones, with their trusty flashlights, back then. "Please..." I begged the owner. "Just let me do 3 sets. You can spot me!" I almost had him convinced too.

Over the years, inclines have always served me well. I was never all that remarkably strong on flat bench presses but inclines were a different story. I reached my lifetime best at the age of 42, pressing 260 pounds for 5 reps, at a body weight of 200 pounds. It wasn't a world record or anything like that but I was really pleased with that accomplishment nonetheless. I attribute my record at age 42 to the following program I developed for inclines. Training chest once per week, it consists of 3 separate workouts. Week one consists of lighter weight and higher reps. For instance, after performing one set of 10 reps with an empty, 45 pound bar, I perform two progressively heavier sets for 10 reps each, followed by one work set with a weight I can perform 15 or more reps with. Week two is the intermediate week where, after performing one set of 10 reps with an empty, 45 pound bar, I perform two progressively heavier sets for 8 reps each, followed by one work set with a weight I can perform 8-9 reps with. Week three consists of our heaviest weights and lowest rep counts. For instance, after performing one set of 10 reps with an empty, 45 pound bar, I perform two progressively heavier sets for 5 reps each, followed by one work set with a weight I can perform 5-6 reps with. Week four goes back to the lighter weight and higher reps and the whole sequence starts over again.

Here's how that might look in a training journal:
Week one:
- Inclines:
- (45) 1X10

- (135, 185) 2X10
- (185) 1X15

Week two:
- Inclines:
- (45) 1X10
- (135, 185) 2X8
- (225) 1X8

Week three:
- Inclines:
- (45) 1X10
- (135, 185) 2X5
- (235) 1X5

Week four:
- start rotation over anew

I recently returned to this same rotation in my training, in 2018, and at the age of 54, incline pressed 237 pounds for 5 reps, at a body weight of 178 pounds.

When performing incline presses, on my way to reaching my lifetime best at age 42, I always followed a strict set-up protocol before each set. I used to carry an index card with me, in my workout journal, that had these 5 steps written on it, for handy reference:

1. Set feet firmly on floor, flat. "Anchor" them in place.
2. Arch lower back slightly.

3. Raise ribcage high.
4. Squeeze scapulae together.
5. Pull shoulders downward (along angle of bench) and push them into the bench.
- Keep tight and set from your toes all the way up to your head.

The actual execution of each rep looked like this:
- elbows wide and under the bar
- forearms perpendicular to the bar
- thumbs wrapped completely around the bar so that you can control it if it starts to drift forward; no false grips allowed
- lower bar to where it just barely clears your chin
- always touch bar to chest, high on chest, every rep
- think SPEED on ascent
- I perform my own lift-offs; it helps lock my shoulders in place
- I always have the spotter help me back onto racks when done

The only difference between how I performed them at age 42 and how I perform them now is that I no longer anchor my feet, in an effort to keep the stress off of my lower back.

This same 3-way rotation can be applied to any compound movement like squats, leg presses, rows and so forth.

Chapter 5

Body Drag Curls

If you keep on doing what you've always done
you'll keep on getting what you've already gotten.
Unknown

"What are you training today?" I said to Danny, as
we both converged on the gym that afternoon. "My
arms; they never change though," he said with a sigh
of disappointment. "No matter what I do, they don't
grow. They haven't grown any in years." Danny's
frustration was palpable. I don't offer advice very
often; most people don't seem to really want it as
much as they just want a sympathetic ear to
commiserate their misfortune to. Nonetheless, I knew
how it felt to be at a sticking point in my training and,
what's more, I had recently discovered a new way to
perform curls that had afforded me significant growth
in my biceps over the past 2 years.

"I used to have the exact same problem as you
Danny. Then, one day, I saw a video where old-time
bodybuilder and trainer to the stars, Vince Gironda,
explained how most bodybuilders have ample
development of the medial head of their biceps
muscle, one of its two heads, but little to no
development of the lateral or outer head." I could see

that Danny was lacking in development of the outer head of his biceps, much like I had been 2 years prior. "Most of the exercises people do for their biceps muscles tend to favor the medial or inner head of the biceps."

I then went on to describe an exercise Vince Gironda was renowned for, body drag curls. "Using a WIDE underhand grip on a barbell, drag it from arms' length upward to where it just touches your chin, never allowing the bar to lose contact with the front of your body AND keeping your elbows back, never allowing them to move forward. It's an awkward feeling movement at first, radically different from traditional curls." "I already work those," Danny interrupted. "Jake, the local trainer, always had me turning my wrist up," demonstrating full supination to me, "whenever we did our dumbbell curls." And, with that, Danny went on his merry, no further arm growth, way.

I have added noticeable size and quality development to my biceps, in my early 50s, from incorporating this one new exercise, after nearly 40 years of weight training. If only Danny's story was the exception. Everybody I've shared this story with has listened semi-politely and then proceeded to tell me how they already incorporated this principle (basis behind body drag curls) in what they are already doing and without ever trying the new exercise. And their arms remain unchanged as a result.

The Reach for the Ring

Chapter 6

Starting Over

This is the test of manhood: How much
is there left in you after you have
lost everything outside yourself.
Orison Swett Marden

Lifting weights is the perfect metaphor for, and mirror of, life: those who want to train will always find a way, regardless of any illness, injury or unforeseen circumstance. And, of course, those who don't will always find an excuse, or ten, to justify their lapses. However, while there are some who will tell you that they have never missed a scheduled workout, my 42-year lifting career has not been like that at all, following a jagged trajectory marred more by false starts and new beginnings, over and over again, than anything else. Learning how to start over anew, when things go awry, has truly become second nature to me.

Physiques are the true "shape-shifters" as evidenced by the sheer speed with which a person's strength and physical development can be completely erased by a single illness or injury. Yet, hopefully, whom one has recognized and developed oneself to be on the inside can be totally impervious to such calamity. In other words, once you've learned what you are capable of, how to build some size and strength, even if it all goes away, you can do it over again and again and again, as needed.

In April of 2001, after an eight year hiatus from competitive bodybuilding, I decided to make my return to the stage at the 2001 N.G.A. Can/Am Bodybuilding Championship, a show where I had won 2nd place in the middleweight division back in 1993. During my 8-year absence, I had attended chiropractic college, earned my doctorate degree, started a family and set up private practice. My training had been sporadic, at best, during my 4 years of chiropractic school and then nearly non-existent during the first 2 years I was in practice. Now, I was back in the saddle, training-wise, and ready to reclaim some glory!

Two days out from the show, I was looking pretty good. Next day, though, my abs had kind of disappeared. "I must be holding water," I reasoned, so I stayed up late that night flexing my abs to flush out the excess water spillage before the morning pre-judging. I was not surprised, nor alarmed in the least, when I was stricken with abdominal cramping during the night. By the morning of the competition, after barely getting any sleep whatsoever the night before, I was feeling weak and my legs were rather shaky, so shaky in fact that I decided to myself, "I'd better skip pumping up before pre-judging or I'm not going to have the strength to climb all of those stairs that lead to the stage." "What a lousy time to get hit with the flu!" I thought.

Pre-judging was tough, but manageable. Everything went rapidly downhill from there. I ended up withdrawing from the contest so I could be taken to the hospital instead. Two emergency rooms, 135 miles apart, over the next 24 hours, followed by life-saving surgery another 12 hours later for a burst appendix, accompanied by peritonitis, that had gone septic and my return to "glory" was replaced by near life-ending "gory." As my surgeon told me afterwards, "All that training you did? It's gone, as if you hadn't trained at all." In the blink of an eye, I had gone from peak condition to ground zero.

Starting back to training after my "adventure" was quite an endeavor, marked by a unique array of "Do"s and "Don't"s. For instance,

Don't:

- Don't do abs immediately post-surgery, while still on a morphine drip! I know, this one sounds obvious, but having been in the mode of doing abs daily, while getting ready for the show, and unaware of the 5" open incision running down the middle of my abdomen and, did I mention the morphine drip?

- Don't do too much too soon. When I was released by my surgeon, to resume training, I asked him, "How about abs, calves and arms?" His reply: "How about just light calves and arms to start."

- Don't let anyone else dictate your limits to you. Following my surgery, my doctors told me I would be lucky to ever attain 60% of the condition I was in beforehand. I chose to believe in myself and my untapped future capacity more than in what the experts told me about such.

Do:

- Do be sure to gradually stress the surgical site. Following any major surgery, the body lays down extensive scar tissue. Initially, this scar tissue is a mish-mash of fibers running in all directions, kind of like a spilled canister of

Pick Up Sticks from grade school. Gradually stressing the surgical site causes the scar tissue to align itself along the stress line, in parallel with the contracting muscle fibers. For the first 3 months I was back to working out, I was physically unable to lay on my back because of the way it pulled on my abdominal incision site. So, during those three months, I substituted weighted dips for bench press until the scar tissue had aligned and stretched enough to allow me to completely lay back without any pain or pulling or risk of further injury.

- Do set training goals and give them your all. When I was in High School, I was able to do 10 reps of dips with 100# of weight tied around my waist. I had not done dips very much since high school but, since they were now my primary chest exercise, I set about repeating my prior best.
- Do be patient. I really was at ground zero, training-wise. It took me a full year to regain most of what I had lost.

Training after such a major illness and surgery required focused dedication combined with a compassionate understanding and appreciation for the body I have been given and all that I was asking it to still accomplish. Some things my body just cannot handle anymore. And that's ok. Learning to gently, consistently nudge my body to greatness, rather than bludgeoning it into submission, has been far more productive and rewarding for me.

Chapter 7

Rehab & Prehab

*Only those who will risk going too far can
possibly find out how far one can go.*
T.S. Eliot

I had just gotten over a cold, one that had forced me
to miss going to the gym for an entire week. I thought
to myself, as I approached the loaded bar for my final
set of standing barbell curls, "If I can just match what
I did last time, I won't end up losing anything." I had
been through this before, why should this time be any
different? My target was 6 reps. "One, two,
three...damn, this feels heavy today... four, you can
do this...five...come on, just one more rep...dig deep...
siiixxxx. Ouch! What the hell was that?" I had
successfully completed my 6th rep but, at the top of
the rep, it felt like somebody had just flicked my left
bicep forcefully with their finger. The sensation
calmed down a little and I finished the rest of my
workout without incident. The next day though, my
left bicep was sore and achy.

Instead of getting better, as time went by, my
left bicep soreness worsened and intensified. The first
set of curls would feel like shards of glass tearing
through my bicep, even if I only used an empty bar.

Once I was then past the initial, agonizing set, my endorphins and enkephalins would seemingly kick in, enabling me to train my heavier sets like normal. And, each time I did so, the next day the pain would be a little worse than before. Eventually, the pain got so severe that I became unable to turn the hand crank to roll my car window up and down.

This injury came on just a few months prior to my burst appendix and, even after 6 weeks of complete rest following my life-saving surgery, it persisted long afterwards. The fancy name for it is tenosynovitis. Basically, the outer fibrous sheath surrounding the muscle had become acutely inflamed and the shards of glass-like sensation I felt during the first set each time was the newly formed adhesions ripping free so the muscle could contract. Treatment for the severely acute stage involved seeing a chiropractor who specialized in soft tissue work, specifically Active Release Technique or A.R.T.

Up until the age of 36, I could get away with coming back to training after a week off, regardless of the cause, and seemingly pick up where I left off. Not any more. If I take a week off for any reason at all, even if it was a planned week off and not due to illness, I still have to start back gradually, doing fewer sets and lighter weights, reducing the weights by anywhere from 10-20%, and taking 3-4 weeks to work my way back up to where I was before the week off. If I had done this at the beginning of this story instead of doing what I did, I would have not gotten injured in the first place.

Throughout the rest of this chapter I will offer up various rehab and prehab exercises that I have personally found beneficial in my training.

Outer elbows:

As I have gotten older, my outer elbows have gotten more sensitive to tendonitis when I push myself too hard, particularly with back exercises like pulldowns, chins and rows. Switching to using a neutral grip on these exercises has helped a lot but that tennis elbow still creeps in from time to time.

There is a company called Theraband that makes a product called the Theraband Flexbar Resistance Bar, designed to rehab tennis elbow, where you twist a foam bar in one particular direction and then slowly release it; and it does help some. Using them reminded me of the eccentric portion of reverse curls and wrist roller extensors. Performing these two exercises, with very slow negatives each rep, the only two exercises where I routinely accentuate the negative, ended up working far better for me.

For healthy lateral elbows, I now regularly alternate between them like this:

- week 1 Standing E-Z bar Reverse Curls
- week 2 Wrist Roller - Extensors
- week 3 Standing E-Z bar Cable Reverse Curls
- week 4 Wrist Roller - Extensors

In the case of the reverse curls, I perform 1x15 reps, focusing on very slow negatives every rep. In the case of the wrist roller, I roll the weight up from the floor by rolling the bar upwards and backwards, towards me, to emphasize the extensor muscles. I hold the wrist roller close to my body to preserve my shoulders and roll the weight up and back down, never letting the weight touch the floor at the bottom, for 1x5-6 reps, again focusing on very slow negatives as I unwind the wrist roller. In both exercises, try to feel the burn on the lateral aspect of your proximal radial head or elbow.

Lower back:

In my experience, acute lower back problems are often the result of a weak lower front. Tight hamstrings often play a role here as well. My favorite way of training my lower abs is hanging knee raises, either on a Captain's Chair or by using Ab Originals Ab Straps that can be clipped on to a chinning bar. I perform mine by twisting side-to-side, trying to touch each knee to the corresponding elbow, with a peak contract squeeze at the top of each rep. These are done slowly and controlled with no momentum at all. Additionally, I perform seated

1-leg hurdlers stretches, on a bench using a light Jump Stretch band for resistance, on leg days right after hamstring exercises.

Chronic lower back problems tend to develop into glute inactivation issues where the glute muscles almost behave like a blown fuse and turn off, oftentimes only on one side. When I was younger, I found high rep good mornings to be a sort of panacea for me, enabling me to resume squatting after several years of inability to perform them. At the time, I routinely performed 2x50-70 reps with 65-75 pounds. As I got older, I reached a point where bending over with weight across my back only served to make my feet go numb, so I had to discontinue doing good mornings.

Louie Simmons, of Westside Barbell, developed a machine to rehab his own lower back after he had fractured it. His Reverse Hyper machine works 1000x better than good mornings ever did and it has become my favorite, favorite exercise ever since I discovered it in 2007. If you ever have the opportunity to use one of Louie's machines I highly recommend it. His Ultra Supreme Reverse Hyper model is the one I have and I can honestly say it's the best investment I have ever made in a piece of weight equipment.

Anterior Tibialis muscle:

Twenty years ago, I suffered for a couple of months from right side foot drop following a squatting injury to my lower back. I sought Gonstead specific chiropractic care for the injury and then started my rehab by regularly training my anterior tibialis muscles during my recovery. Weakness or imbalance of these muscles compared to the calf muscles often contributes to shin splints in runners. There are a few really good machines out there that are designed to work the anterior tibialis muscle; mine is a seated design. But you can also train them without any equipment at all by simply hanging your toes off the end of a 2 inch board or gym mat and raising your feet up and down for around 50-100 reps. These are basically the opposite of calf raises as it is the toes that come off of the ground instead of the heels. I train these with every calf workout.

Hiatal hernia:

In 2011, I cinched my lifting belt up tight so I could lift something heavy into the back of a friend's pickup truck. As soon as I did so, I felt my stomach squish upwards. I had developed a mild hiatal hernia 4-5 years earlier following a bad cough, but this was considerably worse. In addition to seeing a chiropractor who was skilled in adjusting my stomach, I started a new daily exercise regimen that helped a lot too. Stretching.com sells a device they call the Breath Builder. It's basically a ping pong ball housed in a plastic cylinder that you move upwards by breathing forcefully through a thin surgical tube. This exercise is excellent for strengthening the diaphragm. I performed this exercise daily for 5 or 6 years and then scaled back to 3x per week ever since, building up to 16 minutes at a time. It's not a miracle cure but it definitely helps. Between the Breath Builder exercises and having my stomach adjusted periodically, I have never had to have my hiatal hernia surgically repaired.

Training while injured:

During the early '90s, I competed in a number of natural bodybuilding competitions. In fact, between the fall of 1991 and the spring of 1993, I competed every 6 months. The N.G.A. Can/Am Bodybuilding Championship, that I competed in during the spring of 1993, was particularly important to me. I had won my weight class the previous fall at the N.G.A. Buffalo Classic and I was hoping to move up to the next level and win an overall title. Furthermore, this was going to be my final competition before I left for Chiropractic school. Four months out from the competition, I fractured my right hand and had to have my right arm casted up to the elbow. Rather than give up on my plans for competing, I found a way to continue my training. I was unable to grasp anything with my right hand because of the cast, so I had to improvise. I strapped an ankle cuff around my cast and attached it to the crossover machine. This enabled me to perform cable crossovers, lateral raises, triceps pushdowns, curls and one-arm rows. The lighter training volume did my body good allowing me to reach my all-time peak. The picture on the back cover of this book is from that show.

Shoulders:

I have been fortunate to have healthy shoulders throughout my training career. Part of that, no doubt, is due to my meticulous attention to proper form and regular chiropractic care. As I have gotten older, I have made prehab shoulder exercises an integral part of my shoulder training too. Most people, after years of weight training, end up with tight internal rotators and weak external rotators. I regularly stretch my internal rotators for 30-60 seconds at a time, from multiple angles, following all heavy chest and back exercises. Then, to strengthen my external rotators, I perform side-lying flys or side-lying "L" flys, alternating week to week, for 1x20 each arm at the end of my shoulder workout. You can learn more about these exercises by checking out The 7-minute Rotator Cuff Solution, a book by Jerry Robinson and Joseph Horrigan.

Inner Elbows:

A lot of trainees experience pain on the insides of their elbows when they perform triceps exercises, particularly skull krushers. I have found that I can avoid this by training my biceps, at least one exercise for them, prior to training my triceps. Doing so warms my elbows up ahead of time and the added biceps pump seems to cushion my elbows during the subsequent triceps work.

Similarly, I have found that training my hamstrings, performing my leg curls, prior to training my quads with leg presses, warms up my knees ahead of time and the added hamstring pump seems to cushion my knees somewhat during heavier quad work.

Two final points:
Whether training around an injury or just trying to maximize your symmetry, when training alternate limbs with dumbells or cables, I have found it best to always initiate the exercise with the weaker side first, allowing that limb to dictate where the set ends instead of starting with your stronger or dominant limb and potentially training it more than the opposite limb.

Additionally, after suffering from years of lower back issues, I have learned to pre-set my lower back on all standing exercises. What this means is that I flex my glutes strongly and keep my hips tucked forward, or under me, throughout all standing exercises. This really takes all of the stress off of my lower back, preserving it.

The Reach for the Ring

Chapter 8

Spotting Fails

I have made mistakes, but I have never made the
mistake of claiming that I never made one.
James Gordon Bennett, Sr.

The Mummy

"Hey, can you give me a spot?" "Oh, no! It's him again! I hate spotting him. He always makes me do all of the lifting for him," I thought to myself. The rest of us looked at each other with panic and disdain in our eyes, none of us wanting to step forward. "Sure!" I finally said aloud, as I walked towards the bench.

Standing there before me, he looked a bit like an Egyptian mummy, in late 1980's fashion. In addition to wearing the large, print baggy pants and a loose-fitting rag top over a string tank top, like were popular at the time, he was adorned with neoprene elbow sleeves and elastic wrist wraps that dangled loosely at the ends, like a mummy coming undone.

"Keep your hands on the bar at all times," he instructed me. "Only help me if I need it." He struggled from the very first rep with 225 pounds but continued his set for 10 reps. Afterwards, he loaded another pair of 45s onto the bar. "Holy shit bro, you didn't get any reps by yourself with the last set. And now you're gonna go up another 90 pounds?!? Why not?" I screamed inside my head. "Let's go man. You got this!" I said aloud to him. It wasn't a pretty set, more of a set of partial deadlifts for me than a set of bench presses for him, 8 reps worth. My lower back was not amused.

Saddest of all was when the mummy entered a bodybuilding contest about a year later. His arms and legs were impressive, quite formidable in fact. But, his chest development was nearly nonexistent and certainly not up to par with the amount of weight he imagined himself to be pressing.

It's so important to lift your own weights and to "help" others do the same. If you're going to have a spotter assist you with completing a rep, save it for your very last rep of your very last set and, even that, not every workout. Always keep a little reserve in your gas tank. Training to failure and beyond is extremely taxing on the nervous system and more than most people can adequately recover from on a regular basis without the aid of steroids. Personally, I do all of my own liftoffs and all of my own reps always, using a spotter for safety purposes only, just in case, to help guide the weight back onto the rack at the end of a set.

Can you hear me now?

It might be difficult to fathom, in today's day and age, just how spartan the weight room facilities were in universities all across the country as recently as the mid 1980s, when I attended undergraduate studies at Saint Bonaventure University. Weight lifting for athletes had not yet caught on, en masse, out of misplaced fears of making athletes musclebound and slow. So, while the Division I basketball team there had their own private workout room, consisting of relatively useless air shock resistance machines, the rest of us were relegated to an old storage closet, literally, with nothing more than an Olympic bench press bench, an old Universal multi-station machine and a pair of individual squat stands that a prior student had donated. Those of us who wanted dumbbells to workout with brought our own.

Finally, leading into my senior year, the school approved the purchase of a multi-pegged squat rack with safety racks, an incline bench and a seated military press bench. Coming back to school after summer break, but prior to the arrival of the new equipment, conditions were still sparse. Making the change back to such paucity, after having squatted all summer in a tiered step squat rack, with mirrors even, was challenging to say the least. While I had never had to bail from a squat weight before, having learned how to squat from a couple of high level powerlifters, I was familiar with the concept should the need ever arise.

My first squat workout back to school went off without incident: relatively light weights for higher reps. But, squatting without the benefit of safety racks, and with no mirrors or other visual cues to measure depth by, left me feeling uneasy. So, my next workout, where I was scheduled to go heavier for lower reps, I found myself experiencing considerably higher levels of pre-squat jitters than usual.

Franco (not his real name), had volunteered to spot me. He was an experienced, strong lifter who I felt confident in being spotted by. Nonetheless, before starting my heaviest set, I said to him, "Franco, I'm having trouble feeling the proper depth on these today. If I get stuck, just pull it off of me." I then demonstrated to him how to quickly pull the bar back and downwards, should the need arise; and he assured me he understood.

Taking 365 pounds from the wobbly racks, I stepped back and got myself set in position, with Franco standing squarely behind me. As I lowered myself downward, I quickly realized I had descended much too deeply. "Franco, get it off me," I stated. "I got you man; come on," he replied. Panic started to settle in, "Franco, get it off me!" I struggled out again. "No, I got you man. You got this!" But, I knew I didn't. I couldn't. And so, I let go of the bar, dropped my arms and stepped forward as forcefully as I could. Slowly, the bar began to travel down my back, rolling vertebra-by-vertebra, before becoming hung up on my lifting belt. Then, all at once, it popped free from my belt, jettisoning me forward, as though launching from a cannon, into the wall. There came a thunderous crash and, when I turned around, there was Franco on his back, white as a ghost, with the bar across his neck.

Fortunately, Franco was not injured physically. But, he never spoke to me again. Over the course of the school year, others told me I had "ruined" Franco, that he was never the same after that incident. So many people don't really listen to understand. They spend the time being spoken to mentally rehearsing what they want to say next. For effective communication and safety to take place, listen to understand.

Objects in the Rearview Mirror

When I was in high school, back in the early '80s, I had a pair of gravity boots that were sold by former Mr. Universe, Bill Pearl. This was long before inversion tables came on to the scene. Several of my high school classmates and I would sneak off to the gymnasium before classes began and perform inverted sit-ups, just like Richard Gere had done in the 1980 film American Gigolo. After high school ended, I didn't have much occasion to use my gravity boots as I never seemed to train anywhere where there was a chinning bar available.

Approximately 22 years ago, around 1998 or so, I came across an ad for an exercise equipment company that was now selling gravity boots. This was quite unusual since, after the introduction of inversion tables into the market, gravity boots had kind of faded into oblivion. I quickly ordered myself a new pair. As I excitedly awaited their arrival, I went out and purchased a self-standing power tower from the local department store, Montgomery Wards, so that I would have a chinning bar to hang upside down from.

When they arrived, I could barely contain my excitement. Using gravity boots had always made my lower back feel so good. I ran downstairs to my basement gym and strapped the gravity boots around my ankles. "This is going to be so awesome!" I thought to myself. I stretched my arms up to the chinning bar and took hold of it, curled my knees up to my chest, raised my feet above my head, hooked my new gravity boots around the chinning bar and slowly lowered my upper body downwards into full inversion, "Ahhh." It felt exactly like I remembered it... that is, until I tried to get back down! "Oh, shit. I'm stuck!!!" Try as I may, I couldn't curl my upper body up high enough to reach the chinning bar with my hands so I could unhook and get back down. Frantically, I called to my wife who was upstairs in the kitchen making dinner. Words cannot adequately convey the frenzied pandemonium that ensued as my wife, pregnant with our daughter, had to help curl my upper body up high enough for me to reach the chinning bar with my hands so that I could dismount. "What would you have done if I wasn't home to rescue you? You could have died!" she scolded. Maybe it was because of the many lower back injuries I had over the years, maybe it was because I was 40 pounds heavier than I was in high school and maybe it was just because I was 15 years older than the last time I had used gravity boots; whatever the reason, I didn't object when she took my boots away from me.

As a side note, I did start using my gravity boots again about 10 years ago, but this time, I keep a set of Ironmind daisy chains tied to the chinning bar to help me pull myself up enough so that I can get back down without getting stuck.

The Reach for the Ring

Chapter 9

Character Assessment

You can learn more about a person in an hour
of play than in a year of conversation.
Plato

Working out, and going to the gym, has provided me with a lifelong sense of purpose, a never-ending pursuit of excellence. It has given my life structure, a sense of schedule to be followed, even on weekends and holidays, a reason to not drink in excess even during my college years and a reason to eat well. Going to the gym has also provided me with the ultimate screening tool for assessing a person's character. I would venture to say that I have trained in well over 100 gyms across the country over the past 42 years. Whenever I have had to move to a new city for work or school, the gym has always afforded me a means for making new friends and social interaction. All of my closest friendships throughout the years have been forged over the shared common thread of a love for the gym.

You can learn so much from working out with someone:

- What are their goals? And what is their plan for accomplishing them?

- Do they have a plan and stick to it? Or do they change their plan constantly? Do they miss frequently? Do they make excuses?
- What is the level of their commitment?
- How focused are they? Are they easily distracted? Always playing on their phone?
- How do they measure or assess their progress?
- Is there any logic to their training plan? Who designed it? Do they follow trends? How knowledgeable are they?
- Who are they trying to beat? Are they competing with others or with just themselves?
- What kinds of results have they accomplished so far? What was their starting point?
- How hard do they train themselves?
- How open are they to suggestion? Do they already have all the answers or are they perpetual students?
- What kind of form do they train with? Is it sloppy? Reckless? Do they cheat themselves?
- How willing are they to assist you with a spot?

- Are they willing to teach you if you ask them a question?
- How do they treat other gym members: those not as accomplished as them? Those more accomplished than them? Those with conflicting training methodologies or goals? Do they show the same level of respect to all or only to select members and groups?
- Are they braggarts? Full of ego? Do they care about others?
- How do they treat the gym staff?
- How do they treat the gym equipment?
- Do they leave the gym in as good or better condition as they found it? Do they put their weights away when they are done with them? Do they put away weights left behind by others?

As a general rule, I have found that how people do anything is typically how they do everything!

One of the places I loved to train, early in my career, was Bill Knapp's garage gym. Mr. Knapp was a mountain of a man, a steelworker by trade, with a large family and a huge heart to match his phenomenal size and strength. His garage gym was packed full with all of the essential weight equipment one could ask for: an Olympic bench press, a multi-pegged squat rack, a plate-loaded lat pulldown, a stand-up arm-wrestling table, one Olympic bar and tons and tons of weight! Mr. Knapp left his garage open for anyone who wanted to train there.

I arrived there to train legs one day during the summer of 1984. Finding the place empty, I set about my program at the time, 100 crunches to warm up my core, to be immediately followed by barbell back squats. I set the barbell up on the squat rack, loaded it to 135 pounds, then laid down directly beside the squat rack and began my crunches. I was approximately half way done with my set of crunches when Mac Nutello (not his real name) arrived and immediately began stripping the weights off of the bar I had previously set up on the squat rack. While still performing my crunches, I tried explaining to Mac that, while he was welcome to share the bar with me, I was currently using it. He continued stripping the bar down and moved it over to the bench press, telling me, "You're going to have to wait until I'm done with it. I'm not going to be moving it back and forth between sets." Mac was considerably bigger than me at the time and there was nobody else to turn to. I didn't want to cause a scene and then not be allowed to train there again. So, after I finished my crunches I left, enraged that my workout had been so rudely interrupted.

Everybody in the gym has their own reasons for being there. No one's reason is any better or more important than anyone else's. Wipe down machines and benches after each use, re-rack your weights when you are finished with them and, most importantly of all, don't be an asshole!

The Reach for the Ring

Chapter 10

Benefits of a Home Gym

*Different men seek after happiness in
different ways and by different means, and so
make for themselves different modes of life.*
Aristotle

As I mentioned before, I have trained at over 100
gyms throughout the course of my 42 years in weight
training. During this time I have also built two
separate home gyms. When I first got into training,
back in 1978, there were no commercial gyms where
I lived, only the local Y.M.C.A., which I found quite
intimidating at the time. So I built a small home gym
of my own that started out with a sleeping bag draped
across an old coffee table with iron legs and wooden
top for my bench and an Ultra-K-tron plastic 110-
pound weight set. Throughout my high school years
my home gym grew to ultimately include several
pieces from Ed Jubinville: a 7-in-1 bench (a multi-
angle bench with a preacher curl attachment, a wrist
curl attachment, and dip bar/squat rack attachments),
an incline/decline bench, a plate loaded lat machine,
a leg extension/leg curl machine, a grip machine and
a hyperextension bench. There was also an inverted
leg press from Dan Lurie and nearly 1000 pounds of
mostly York weights. I sold all of it after my

freshman year of college, but I always knew that someday I would build another.

After completing Chiropractic school in 1996, I again set about accumulating equipment for a home gym. This time, there were commercial gyms, which I also trained at. But I wanted a home set-up as well so that I could continue my training while not being absent from my family. Over the next 20+ years, I accumulated a massive amount of equipment for my home gym, this time mostly from Ed Jubinville's son, Robert.

There are many benefits to having a home gym. Here's just a sampling:

- Open (available) 24 hours per day, 7 days per week, year round, including holidays.
- Never have to wait for a piece of equipment to become available. If you have ever trained at a commercial gym and tried to access a bench on Monday afternoon, or any piece of equipment the first 3 weeks of January, you know what I am talking about here.
- 100% control over music type AND volume.
- Stocked with exactly the pieces of equipment I would choose if I were

setting up my ideal gym. (always a work in progress)

- No wasted time and gas driving to/from gym.
- No bonehead rules to follow. (This one is big!) Rules like no chalk, no dropping the weights, no screaming during sets (an actual rule at a Gold's Gym I once worked at. Seriously! A friend of mine got kicked out for doing it.), no posing in the gym (also an actual rule at the Gold's where I worked. I was allotted special permission to pose, because I was competing at the time, so long as I only posed in the men's locker room. What could go wrong?!?).
- No bonehead members to deal with: bullies, chatterboxes, equipment hogs, sweat factories without towels, Don Juans, know-it-alls, infectious doses, people playing on their phones.
- No annual dues. Money saved can be invested in more equipment.
- Allows for more creativity in workouts: can set up circuits, giant sets, etc. involving multiple pieces of equipment, without infringing upon others' workouts. Can take workouts outside in good weather.

- It's just plain fun!
- Much cleaner locker rooms and toilets!
- No dress codes.
- No need to wear a mask during pandemics like Covid 19.

I realize not everyone has the space or the money to set up a home gym, but for those who can, I highly recommend it. Start by getting just enough equipment to train one body part, or one training day, e.g. chest, shoulders and triceps. Some creative ways to get started could include having several people work together, perhaps each accumulating enough equipment for one different body part; for instance, one person could gather leg equipment, another could gather chest equipment and a third could gather back equipment. Then you would each have 3 different gyms to train at! Some people build a "man cave" for their entertainment needs, some have extra garages for their cars. For me, I'll take a fully stocked home gym every day of the week!

Chapter 11

Rotations & Routines

*Persistent people begin their success
where others end in failure.*
Edward Eggleston

Everything you will read in this chapter comes
directly from my training journals, which I have
meticulously kept throughout the years. In some
cases you will notice unusual weight amounts. This is
because I primarily use standard weights instead of
Olympic weights in my home gym and the bars start
out at 32 pounds instead of 45 pounds like you are
used to. In all cases, the weights listed are actual.

The first rotation I want to share is taken from
my pre-contest preparations for the 1992 N.G.A.
Can/Am. I experimented with an unusual training
methodology for this particular show and the results
make it worthy of mention. As a general rule, most
people are not able to add muscular size while dieting
down for competition, not naturally anyway. Rather,
dieting down for show is usually a delicate balance as
you try to shed body fat while retaining as much of
your hard earned muscle as possible. Keeping your
muscle mass can be tricky. Your joints are no longer
padded with a layer of fat and they tend to get more

easily irritated by heavy weights now. And yet, you need to keep your strength up so that you don't lose size.

I had just learned about this particular training methodology in the final weeks leading up to my previous show, the A.N.B.C. Natural Westmoreland and I wanted to try it out for the entire 10 weeks of pre-contest prep. The training sequence was such that it called for training three days on, followed by one day off, and splitting the body into three separate workouts. The thing that made it unique was this: the rest periods. Rest between sets was strictly limited to 20 seconds. Every set of every exercise was done with only a 20 second break between them. Regular rest periods could be taken between exercises. In order to make this doable, all weights were limited to 70% of my usual working weights. As the show got closer, maintaining these weights became ever more challenging. However, because the weights weren't really all that heavy to begin with, the risk of injury was low and my joints were not overtaxed.

I can honestly say that this particular program resulted in my absolute tightest, lowest body fat condition ever, albeit certainly not my biggest.

For each exercise, after the first set was completed, the weight was set down and I counted silently in my head "one one-thousand, two one-thousand..." all the way up to "twenty one-thousand." And then the weight was picked back up and the next set commenced.

The Reach for the Ring

Day 1A (3/21/1992)

Incline Press (155) 5X8
- 20 second rests btwn sets

Supine db Flys (50) 4X12,12,12,11
(45) 1X12
- 20 second rests btwn sets

Top Cable Crossovers (50) 4X15
- 20 second rests btwn sets

Seated BB French Press (65) 5X10
- 20 second rests btwn sets

V-Bar Tricep Pushdowns (60) 5X12
- 20 second rests btwn sets

Seated Alternate db Press (35) 5X12
- 20 second rests btwn sets

Standing db Lateral Raises (15) 4X10
- 20 second rests btwn sets

Partial Sit-ups 4X20
- regular rests btwn sets
- arms across chest

note: Practiced 60 second poses for chest and triceps

Day 2A (3/22/1992)

Nautilus Leg Extensions (90) 5X12
- 20 second rests btwn sets

Hack Squats (60) 5X10
- 20 second rests btwn sets
- feet and knees together

Seated Toe Raise (60) 3X15
          (50) 3X15
- 20 second rests btwn sets

Standing Calf Raise (70) 5X15
- 20 second rests btwn sets

note: Practiced 60 second poses for legs

Day 3A (3/23/1992)

Supported Rows (70) 5X10
- 20 second rests btwn sets

Parallel Close Grip Pulldowns (140) 5X10
- 20 second rests btwn sets

Seated Chest Lat Pulldowns (130) 4X10
- 20 second rests btwn sets

BB Shrugs (225) 3X13
- 20 second rests btwn sets

Standing BB Curls (80) 4X8
(75) 1X8
- 20 second rests btwn sets

Seated Alternate db Curls (30) 4X12
- 20 second rests btwn sets

Kneeling BB Wrist Curls (45) 3X20,15,10
- 20 second rests btwn sets

Prone Leg Curls (50) 5X10
- 20 second rests btwn sets

BB Good Mornings (35) 2X75
- regulars rests btwn sets

Crunches (0) 3X25 supersetted with
Twisting Alternate Knee-ins 3X25
- regular rests btwn sets

Practiced 60 sec. poses for back & biceps

Day 1B (3/25/1992)

Incline Press (155) 5X8
- 20 second rests btwn sets

Supine db Flys (50) 4X12
(45) 1X12
- 20 second rests btwn sets

Top Cable Crossovers (30) 4X15
- 20 second rests btwn sets

Seated BB French Press (70) 5X10
- 20 second rests btwn sets

V-Bar Tricep Pushdowns (60) 5X12
- 20 second rests btwn sets

Seated Alternate db Press (35) 5X12
- 20 second rests btwn sets

Standing db Lateral Raises (15) 4X10
- 20 second rests btwn sets

Partial Sit-ups 4X20
- regular rests btwn sets
- arms across chest

note: Practiced 60 second poses for chest and triceps

Day 2B (3/26/1992)

Nautilus Leg Extensions (90) 5X12
- 20 second rests btwn sets

BB Back Squats (135,155,175,175,185) 5X10
- regular rests btwn sets

Angled Leg Press (90,180,200,200,200) 5X10
- regular rests btwn sets

Seated Toe Raise (60) 4X15
(50) 2X15
- 20 second rests btwn sets

Standing Calf Raise (70) 5X15
- 20 second rests btwn sets

note: Practiced 60 second poses for legs

Day 3B (3/27/1992)

Supported Rows (70) 5X10
  * 20 second rests btwn sets
Parallel Close Grip Pulldowns (140) 5X10
  * 20 second rests btwn sets
Seated Chest Lat Pulldowns (130) 4X10
  * 20 second rests btwn sets
BB Shrugs (225) 3X13
  * 20 second rests btwn sets

Standing BB Curls (80) 4X8
                 (75) 1X8
  * 20 second rests btwn sets
Seated Alternate db Curls (30) 4X12
  * 20 second rests btwn sets
Reverse BB Curls (45) 3X10
  * 20 second rests btwn sets

Prone Leg Curls (50) 5X10
  * 20 second rests btwn sets
BB Good Mornings (35) 2X75
  * regulars rests btwn sets

Crunches (0) 3X25 supersetted with
Twisting Alternate Knee-ins 3X25
  * regular rests btwn sets
Practiced 60 sec. poses for back & biceps

This next rotation is taken from my preparation for the 1992 N.G.A. Buffalo Classic. This training sequence still called for training three days on, followed by one day off, and splitting the body into three separate workouts. There were two pretty big differences this time compared to my training for the '92 Can/Am. This time, I eliminated the 20 second rest time limits on all but a select few isolation movements. Furthermore, I developed four separate leg day programs. I will share with you here one complete rotation as well as all four separate leg day routines. Also, I switched gyms around this time, hence the difference in weight used on the leg press. All leg presses are not the same.

Day 1 (10/10/1992) - Leg Day #1

Angled Leg Press (0) 1X12
            (180,210,230,250,260)
            5X10,10,10,10,9
        • feet straight, close (3" apart)
Leg Extensions (70) 3X15
            (80) 1X15

Seated Toe Raise Machine (60,70,80,90,90)
            5X12,12,12,10,10
Standing 1-Leg db Toe Raise (45)
            5X12,12,11,11,10

note: Practiced 60 second poses for legs and calves

<u>Day 2 (10/11/1992)</u>

Parallel Close Grip Pulldowns to Chest
　　　　　(150,170,190,200,180)
　　　　　5X10
Seated Chest Lat Pulldowns (150,170,170,170)
　　　　　4X10
BB Bentover Rows (150) 2X12 Wide Grip
　　　　　　　　(150) 2X12 Close Grip
　　　　　• overhand grip on all sets
BB Shrugs (225) 3X12

Standing BB Curls (65,75,80,80) 4X15
Seated Alternate db Curls (35) 4X12
　　　　　　• 20 second rests btwn sets
Kneeling BB Wrist Curls (55) 3X20

BB Good Mornings (65) 2X50
Prone Leg Curls (70) 4X12

note: Practiced 60 second poses for back, traps
and biceps

<u>Day 3 (10/12/1992)</u>

Incline Press (135,185,205,215,215)
       5X8,8,8,6,5
Supine db Flys (50) 5X12
       • 20 second rests btwn sets
Top Cable Crossovers (65) 5X12
       • 20 second rests btwn sets

Seated BB Press Behind-the-Neck
       (95,115,135,145,145)
       5X10,10,10,8,7
Standing db Lateral Raises (25) 3X12
Standing Alternate db Front Raise (20,20,15)
       3X12
       • supersetted together

EZ Skull Krushers (65,70,70,70,65) 5X12
V-Rope Tricep Pushdowns (40,40,35,35)
       4X12
       • 20 second rests btwn sets

Crunches (0) 3X30 supersetted with
Twisting Alternate Knee-ins 3X30

note: Practiced 60 second poses for chest,
shoulders and triceps

<u>Leg Day #2 (10/14/1992)</u>

Back Squats (45) 1X12
        (135,165,185,195,185)
        5X15
Leg Extensions   (70) 2X15
         (60) 2X15

Seated Toe Raise Machine (50,60,70,70,60)
        5X15
Standing 1-Leg db Toe Raise (25) 3X15
                (20) 2X15
note: Practiced 60 second poses for legs and
calves

==

<u>Leg Day #3 (10/18/1992)</u>

Angled Leg Press (90,140,150,160,170)
        5X20
      • feet straight; close (3")
Leg Extensions   (70) 2X15
         (60) 2X15

Seated Toe Raise Machine (50,60,70,70,70)
        5X15
Standing 1-Leg db Toe Raise (25) 3X15
                (20) 2X15

<u>Leg Day #4 (10/22/1992)</u>

Back Squats (45) 1X12
            (135,185,205,225,235)
            5X10,10,10,10,7
Leg Extensions   (70) 2X15
            (60) 2X15

Seated Toe Raise Machine (60,70,80,90,90)
            5X12,12,12,10,10
Standing 1-Leg db Toe Raise (45) 5X12

note: Practiced 60 second poses for legs and
calves

The Reach for the Ring

This particular rotation, taken from my pre-contest prep for the 1993 N.G.A Can/Am, is one of my all-time favorites. I mentioned previously how I was forced to train with a broken hand for about a month leading up to my pre-contest prep for this particular show. In fact, it actually cut my pre-contest prep time short by about two weeks. However, the decreased training volume while my arm was in a cast resulted in considerable gains in muscle size. This made me realize how badly I had been overtraining up to this point and I sought a new rotation to maximize my recovery going forward, even in the face of pre-contest preparation.

I had read in the past about a sequence where the body was still split into three separate workouts but training was done on a three days on, one day off, two days on, one day off rotation. The benefit to this rotation is that the same two days are off week-to-week. Each body part gets worked five times every three weeks. It takes three weeks to cycle completely through and have the same workout occur on the same day of the week.

I decided I wanted still more recovery built into my program than even this allowed. So I opted to continue to split my body into three separate workouts, but on a two days on, one day off rotation. The gyms were open 7 days per week where I was living at the time and my schedule allowed me to train any day of the week I wanted to, so having specific days of the week off was not an issue. Every third week, there were only four training days instead of five. And this rotation allowed me to plan better for certain body parts. For example, leg day: every other leg workout, the two day rotation was started off with leg day; this is the day I chose to do my squats, since I was most rested. Every other leg workout, the two day rotation had leg day fall on the second consecutive day of training; this is the day I chose to do my leg presses.

Using this new rotation of two days on, one day off, while still splitting my body into three separate workouts, enabled me to reach my lifetime best development. Like with the '92 Buffalo Classic, I developed four separate leg day programs. I will share with you here two complete weeks of workouts, including all four separate leg day routines. I trained at several gyms while getting ready for this show so weight variances from one workout to another were, in large part, solely due to using different machines in these different gyms. Four different gyms are represented in this sampling alone.

Day 1 (3/30/1993) Tuesday

BB Back Squats (45) 1X12
(135,185,205,225,240)
5X10,10,10,10,8

Hack Squats   (50,70,80,90,105)
5X10
- heels at 90 degree angle
- heels together

Seated Toe Raise Machine (70,90,100,110,115)
5X12,12,12,10,7

Standing Toe Raise Machine (120/110/100/70/40)
3X12/6/6/6/6
- "tear downs"

note: Practiced 60 second poses for legs

Heavy Squat Day
================

Day 2 (3/31/1993) Wednesday

BB Good Mornings (65) 2X50
Prone Leg Curls (80) 5X15

Seated Chest Lat Pulldowns (150,170,190,200)
                    4X10
Parallel Close Grip Pulldowns to Chest
                    (150,170,170,170)
                    4X10
BB Bentover Rows (150) 2X15 wide grip
                    (150) 2X15 close grip
        •   overhand grip on all sets
BB Shrugs (225) 3X12

Standing BB Curls (65,75,80,80) 4X15
Seated Alternate db Curls (40) 4X12
            •   with twist at top of each rep
Reverse BB Curls (55) 3X12

note: Practiced 60 second poses for back, traps
and biceps

Day 3 (4/2/1993) Friday

Crunches (0) 3X30 supersetted w/
Hanging Knee Raises 3X30

Incline Press (135,185,205,215,195)
                    5X10,10,10,9,10
Supine db Flys (60) 4X12
        • w/ twist at top
Decline db Flys (55) 4X12
        • w/ twist at top

----

1. Standing db Lateral Raises (30) 4X12
2. a.) Standing Alternate db Front Raises (25) 2X
2. b.) Bentover db Lateral Raises (35) 2X
        • supersetted 1. w/ 2.

Kneeling V-Bar Tricep Pushdowns (120) 4X15
Seated BB French Press (45,65,70,75,75)
                    5X12

note: Practiced 60 second poses for chest,
shoulders and triceps

<u>Day 1 (4/3/1993) Saturday</u>

Seated Toe Raise Machine (70,90,110,120,120)
            5X12,12,12,7,6

Standing Toe Raise Machine (130/120/100/70/40)
            3X12/6/6/6/6
        • "tear downs"
Standing Toe Lifts 3X30

Angled Leg Press (0) 1X12
            (180,210,240,260,270)
            5X10,10,10,10,9
        • feet straight; close (3")

Leg Extensions (70) 5X15

note: Practiced 60 second poses for legs

Heavy Leg Press Day
====================

Day 2 (4/5/1993) Monday

BB Good Mornings (65) 2X50
Prone Leg Curls (60) 5X15

Parallel Close Grip Pulldowns to Chest
                    (150,170,190,200)
                    4X10
Seated Chest Lat Pulldowns (150,170,180,180)
                    4X10
BB Bentover Rows (150) 2X15 wide grip
                    (150) 2X15 close grip
          • overhand grip on all sets
BB Shrugs (225) 3X12

Standing BB Curls (65,75,80,80) 4X15
Seated Alternate db Curls (40) 4X12,12,12,16
          • with twist at top of each rep
Kneeling BB Wrist Curls (60) 3X20,20,17

note: Practiced 60 second poses for back, traps
and biceps

Day 3 (4/6/1993) Tuesday

Incline Press (135,185,205,205,195)
                         5X10
               • needed help w/ last rep 4th set
Supine db Flys (60) 4X12
                    • w/ twist at top
Kneeling Top Cable Crossovers (80) 4X12

Standing db Lateral Raises (30) 4X12
Seated Shoulder Press Machine (65,65,55,55)
                         4x12
               • supersetted together

Kneeling V-Bar Tricep Pushdowns (120) 4X15
                    • crossover unit
EZ Skull Krushers (65) 5X12

Crunches (0) 3X30 supersetted w/
Seated Knee-ins 3X30

note Practiced 60 second poses for chest,
shoulders and triceps

<u>Day 1 (4/8/1993) Thursday</u>

BB Back Squats   (45) 1X12
                   (135,165,185,210,185)
                   5X15

Hack Squats   (40,60,70,70,60)
                   5X15
- heels at 90 degree angle
- heels together

Seated Toe Raise Machine (70,90,110,120,115)
                   5X12,12,12,7,7

Standing Toe Raise Machine (130) 5X12

note: Practiced 60 second poses for legs

High Rep Light Squat Day
=======================

<u>Day 2 (4/9/1993) Friday</u>

BB Good Mornings (65) 2X50
Nautilus Prone Leg Curls (D,E,E,E,E) 5X15

Seated Chest Lat Pulldowns (150,170,190,200)
                    4X10
Parallel Close Grip Pulldowns to Chest
                    (150,170,170,170)
                    4X10
BB Bentover Rows (150) 2X15 wide grip
                    (150) 2X15 close grip
            •   overhand grip on all sets
BB Shrugs (225) 3X12

Standing BB Curls (65,75,80.5,80.5) 4X15
Seated Alternate db Curls (40) 4X12,12,12,16
Reverse BB Curls (55) 3X12

note: Practiced 60 second poses for back, traps
and biceps

Day 3 (4/11/1993) Sunday

Crunches (0) 3X30 supersetted w/
Twisting Alternate Knee-ins 3X30

Incline Press (135,185,205,215,195)
5X10,10,10,9,10
  • needed help w/ last rep 4th set
Supine db Flys (60) 4X12
  • w/ twist at top
Decline db Flys (55) 4X12
  • w/ twist at top

----

1. Standing db Lateral Raises (30) 4X12
2. a.) Standing Alternate db Front Raises (25) 2X
2. b.) Bentover db Lateral Raises (35) 2X
  • supersetted 1. w/ 2.

Kneeling V-Bar Tricep Pushdowns (45) 4X15
Wide Grip BB Skull Krushers (45,65,65,65,70.5)
5X12

note: Practiced 60 second poses for chest,
shoulders and triceps

Day 1 (4/12/1993) Monday

Seated Toe Raise Unit (95,110,120,130,130)
             5X12,12,12,8,8

Smith Machine Standing Toe Raise
             (50,90,140,140,140)
             5X12

Angled Leg Press (0) 1X12
             (90,140,180,210,210)
             5X20
        • feet straight; close (1")

Nautilus Leg Extensions (F,G,G,H,H) 5X15

Standing Toe Lifts 3X30

note: Practiced 60 second poses for legs

High Rep Light Leg Press Day
============================

This next sequence is based on a two-week rotation that I enjoyed following back in February of 2000. As I reached my mid-30s, my need for longer periods of recovery between workouts increased. Each major body part gets trained three times every two weeks and it has the same days off from training each week. It goes like this:

- Day 1 Lower Body (Saturday)
- Day 2 Upper Body (Sunday)
- Day 3 Rest (Monday)
- Day 4 Back, Biceps, Forearms (Tuesday)
- Day 5 Rest (Wednesday)
- Day 6 Legs (Thursday)
- Day 7 Rest (Friday)
- Day 8 Chest, Shoulders, Triceps (Saturday)
- Day 9 Back, Biceps, Forearms (Sunday)
- Day 10 Rest (Monday)
- Day 11 Legs (Tuesday)
- Day 12 Rest (Wednesday)
- Day 13 Chest, Shoulders, Triceps (Thursday)
- Day 14 Rest (Friday)

The Reach for the Ring

Day 1 (Saturday)

BB Good Mornings (25,40) 2X55

Standing 1-Leg Curls (60,60,50) 3X12

Hip Belt Squats (60,80,110,110)
          4X10,10,15,15

Moon Bench db Pullovers (20) 2X20

      • done immediately after last 2 sets of
        squats

Seated Toe Raises (65) 3X15

      • 3 second pause at top

Sissy Squats (10) 3X15

Donkey Calf Raises (170) 2X20

Day 2 (Sunday)

Incline db Press (60) 3X10
- 30 second rest btwn sets

1-Arm db Rows (55) 3X15
- no rest btwn sets

Standing db Lateral Raises (15) 3X12
- 30 second rest btwn sets

Incline Alternate db Curls (30) 3X12,12,8
- 30 second rest btwn sets

Seated Knee-ins on Bench 2X30
Crunches 2X20

Day 4 (Tuesday)

Hyperextensions 1X20
BB Bentover Rows (141) 4X15
- underhand grip

BB Shrugs (141) 3X13

Standing BB Curls (75,90,90,95) 4X8
Seated 1-Arm db Concentration Curls
(25) 3X12

Bent-knee Leg Raises 2X20
Crunches w/ legs over bench 2X15

Day 6 (Thursday)

BB Good Mornings (40,45) 2X55
Standing 1-Leg Curls (60) 3X12

Hip Belt Squats (60,80,110,110)
        4X10,10,20,20
Moon Bench db Pullovers (20) 2X20
- done immediately after last 2 sets of squats

Seated Toe Raises (65) 3X15
- 3 second pause at top

Sissy Squats (10) 3X15
Donkey Calf Raises (170) 2X20

Day 8 (Saturday)

Incline Press (132,182,202,202) 4X10
Supine db Flys (45) 3X12

Seated Alternate db Press (45) 4X10
Standing db Lateral Raises (25) 2X12

Skull Krushers (60,60,60,70) 4X12

Seated Knee-ins on Bench 2X30
Crunches 2X20

Day 9 (Sunday)

Hyperextensions 1X20
BB Bentover Rows (141) 4X15
* underhand grip
BB Shrugs (141) 3X13

Standing BB Curls (75,90,95,95) 4X8
Seated EZ Preacher Curls (60) 2X12
* close grip

Seated BB Wrist Curls (55) 2X15

Ab Wheel 2X20

Day 11 (Tuesday)

BB Good Mornings (45) 2X55
Standing 1-Leg Curls (60) 3X12

Hip Belt Squats (60,80,110,110)
        4X10,10,20,20
Moon Bench db Pullovers (20) 2X20
        • done immediately after last 2 sets of
          squats
Seated Toe Raises (65) 3X15
        • 3 second pause at top
Sissy Squats (10) 3X15
Donkey Calf Raises (170) 3X20

Day 13 (Thursday)

Incline Press (132,182,202,202) 4X10
Supine db Flys (50) 3X12

Seated Alternate db Press (50) 4X10
Standing db Lateral Raises (25) 2X12

Skull Krushers (60,70,70,80) 4X12

Seated Knee-ins on Bench 2X30
Crunches 2X20

When I was released by my surgeon to resume my training, following my ruptured appendix in 2001, I asked him, "How about abs, calves and arms?" His reply: "How about just light calves and arms to start." Here now are those very first two workouts, my training sequence seven weeks later and, finally, my training sequence seven months later so you can see my progress.

First Workout Post-Surgery (06/12/2001)

Standing Calf Raise (405) 3X10,10,8 1/2
Seated Tibial Raise (15) 2X15

Standing BB Curls (75) 3X8

Standing Back Wrist Curls (65) 2X15

====================================

Second Workout Post-Surgery (06/14/2001)

Dips (0) 3X12

Standing db Lateral Raises (15) 2X12

<u>Seven Weeks Later Post-Surgical Release</u>
- 13 week (3 month) surgical anniversary
- 1st time Bench Pressing since surgery

<u>Day 1 (7/30/2001)</u>

Bench Press (45,135,185,185,185)
     5X10

Seated Alternate db Press (55) 3X13,14,12

Supported T-Bar Rows (45,50) 2X15

----

db Reverse Wrist Curls (15) 2X15

Day 2 (8/2/2001)
- 1st time training abs since surgery

Standing Calf Raise (405,465,525,545,465)
        5X10,10,8 1/2,6 1/2,10
Seated Tibial Raise (20) 2X15
Seated Toe Raise (80) 1X17

Standing BB Curls (75,90,102.5,102.5)
        4X8
Seated EZ Preacher Curls (70) 2X12,11
- close grip

Standing Back Wrist Curls (80) 2X15

Ab Bench Crunches (15) 1X15
Seated Knee-ins 1X25
- ab exercises supersetted together

Day 3 (8/4/2001)

Dips (0,12,65,65,65) 5X8

Seated Alternate db Press (60,60,50) 3X13,13,15

Supported T-Bar Rows (50) 2X15

----

db Reverse Wrist Curls (15) 2X15

note: on 8/10/2001, I re-introduced BB Back Squats with (45) 1X15. On 8/16/2001, that went to (45,65,65) 3X5,5,20 breathing-style.

Seven Months Later Post-Surgical Release

Day 1 (1/20/2002)

Hip Belt Squats (60,110,120)
          3X5,5,17
Moon Bench db Pullovers (20) 1X30
     • done immediately after last set of
       squats

Standing Calf Raise (405) 5X15,12,11,10,10

Seated Tibial Raise (21.25) 2X15

Seated Toe Raise (80) 1X17

Ab Wheel 2X35,30

<u>Day 2 (1/24/2002)</u>

Incline Press (45) 1X5
          (135,185,220,205)
          4X10,10,11,10

Supine db Flys (50) 3X13

BB Bentover Rows (100) 2X15 wide grip
               (100) 2X15 medium grip
          • overhand grip on all sets
Hyperextensions 2X20,15

Day 3 (1/26/2002)

Dips (0,15,100,100) 4X8,8,10,8

Standing V-Bar Tricep Pushdowns (80,70)
                                    2X12

Standing BB Curls (75,90,107.5,107.5)
                                    4X8,8,8,6
Seated Alternate db curls (40,35,35)
                                    3X12,12,15

Standing Back Wrist Curls (75,80) 2X15

db Reverse Wrist Curls (12) 2X15

Day 4 (1/27/2002)

BB Back Squats (45,45,151)
                    3X5,5,22 breathing-style
Moon Bench db Pullovers (20) 1X30
- done immediately after last set of squats

Standing Calf Raise (405,465,545,545,465)
                    5X10,10,7,7,9
Seated Tibial Raise (21.25,22.5) 2X15

Seated Toe Raise (80) 1X18

Ab Wheel 1X35

The four-week sequence that follows is my current rotation and routine for 2020. I split my entire body into four separate workouts, training each body part only once per week. As you will see, I have a certain amount of variability built into the program while still focusing on the basics. I alternate between one week with lighter weights and higher reps, and then going heavier with lower reps the following week.

You will recall that earlier in the book I referred to the 3-week rotation that I used to bring my Inclines up to record levels. Eventually, rather than perpetually trying to get stronger on Inclines, I switched to a "working weights" methodology so that I could continue to extract growth from my program without risking injury by training ever heavier. I developed a conversion chart for myself that enables me to move between rep schemes that has worked well for me on Inclines, Rows and Standing Calves. It would likely work on other exercises as well. Here it is:

- 1X26 = 3X15
- 1X20 = 3X12 = 2X15
- 1X16 = 3X10 = 2X12

Basically, if I can perform one set of 20 reps with a given weight, I can likely perform three sets of 12 with that same weight instead, or two sets of 15 with that same weight instead. This enables me to slightly increase my training intensity and volume without overtaxing my joints.

You will also likely notice that the weights I am currently able to use for leg training are relatively light. Life's like that sometimes. Due to the effects of aging, prior injuries, and so on, some things just aren't going to be what they once were. That's why the weights are adjustable. You can always still train, regardless of what your current limitations may be. I know I sure will.

Week One, Day One (Saturday)

Prone Leg Curl (85,105,105) 3X15
- Toes Plantar Flexed (Pointed)
- Peak Contract

Leg Press (0,50,90) 3X10,10,16
- feet straight; close (3.5" apart)
- feet low on platform
- focused on drive through heels ("feel the heels")
- moderate depth, 15 or more rep target
- breathing-style reps 3rd set (3 breaths btwn each rep)

Reverse Hypers-Tilt Forward-With Roller (0+,35+,50+) 3X15,15,25
- Peak Contract
- focused on form, minimizing momentum

Seated 1-leg Hurdler Stretch on Bench 3X each leg
- w/ Jump Stretch Band

Hack Squats (40) 2X12
- Reverse Double Banded
- Heels together, feet at 90 degrees

Standing Thigh/hip flexor stretches 3X each leg

Week One, Day Two (Sunday)

Incline Press (42) 1X10
          (132,182,187,187)
          4X10,10,12,12
- scapulae retracted
- feet <u>not</u> anchored

Standing db lateral raises (17.5) 2X15
- brief pause at top of each rep

Side-lying "L" fly (10) 1X20

Dragon Flags 1X15
- Ab board
- 2nd rung up from top

Ab Wheel - kneeling 1X20

note: performed internal rotator stretches after inclines

<u>Week One, Day Three (Tuesday)</u>

Seated WIDE Grip Chest Lat Pulldowns
          (100,130,130) 3X12,12,15
- Traditional-style bar
- Continuous-style reps

Parallel WIDE Grip KC Rows
          (105,150,150) 3X12,15,15+8 SR
- Pause w/ Peak Contract
- SR=Scapular Retractions

Seated Parallel Close Grip Pulldowns to Chest
          (130) 1X15
- Revolving handle
- continuous-style reps

Seated Toe Raise (80) 3X15
- wide, toes out foot placement
- 1-second pause at top

Standing Tibial Raise 1X50
- heels on mat, toes hanging off
- held onto Incline rack for balance

note: performed internal rotator stretches during rows

note: performed thigh/hip flexor and calf stretches during calves

Week One, Day Four (Thursday)

Seated EZ Preacher Curls (65,75) 2X15
- close grip

Standing V-bar Tricep Pushdowns (70) 1X18
- Lat Machine

Incline db curls (30) 1X15
- Palms up (fully supinated)
- good stretch at bottom

EZ Skull Krushers (65,90) 2X15
- lowered behind head
- scapulae retracted

Standing EZ Reverse Curls (65) 1X15
- knurled grip
- very slow negatives

Wrist Roller--Flexors (40) 1X5

note: all sets and reps done SLOW & STRICT

<u>Week Two, Day One (Saturday)</u>

Prone Leg Curl (85,105,105) 3X15
- Toes Plantar Flexed (Pointed)
- Peak Contract

Leg Extensions (20) 3X12

Banded Walks w/ Bands 1X50

Leg Press-Partials(0,50,90,145) 4X10,10,10,15
- feet straight; close (3.5" apart)
- feet low on platform
- focused on drive through heels ("feel the heels")
- partial depth, <u>15 or more rep target</u>
- breathing-style reps 3rd set (3 breaths btwn each rep)

Reverse Hypers-Tilt Forward-With Roller (0+,35+) 2X15,40
- Peak Contract
- focused on form, minimizing momentum

Seated 1-leg Hurdler Stretch on Bench 3X each leg
- w/ Jump Stretch Band

Standing Thigh/hip flexor stretches 3X each leg

Week Two, Day Two (Sunday)

Decline Press (42) 1X10
(132,182,187,187)
4X12
- scapulae retracted

Supine db flys (46) 2X20
- Peak Contract
- scapulae retracted

Standing db lateral raises (17.5) 2X15
- brief pause at top of each rep

Side-lying fly (10) 1X20

Ab Strap Twisting Knee Raise (0) 1X26
- 13 reps per side
- Pause w/ Peak Contract
- slow & controlled w/o any swing

Ab Bench Crunches (30) 1X20
- Pause w/ Peak Contract

Week Two, Day Three (Tuesday)

Seated Parallel WIDE Grip Chest Lat Pulldowns
(130,150,150) 3X12,12,15
- Wide neutral grip bar
- Continuous-style reps

Parallel WIDE Grip KC Rows
(105,150,150) 3X12,15,15+8 SR
- Pause w/ Peak Contract
- SR=Scapular Retractions

Overhead Strap Pulls (130) 1X15
- leather V-strap
- Pull from close together to diverging

Standing Calf Raises (405) 3X12
- knees locked
- 1-second pause at top

Seated Tibial Raise (32.5) 1X25

note: performed internal rotator stretches during rows
note: performed thigh/hip flexor and calf stretches during calves

Week Two, Day Four (Thursday)

Standing Wide Grip BB Body Drag Curls (65) 2X15
- Thumbs under bar instead of over
- Vince Gironda style

Standing V-Rope Tricep Pushdowns (50) 1X15
- Lat Machine

BB KC Curls (65) 1X15
- Spider curls on Knee-Chest Row Bench
- Pause at top & bottom
- Peak contract at top
- Wide Grip
- Thumbs over bar (wrapped around)

EZ Skull Krushers (65,90) 2X15
- lowered behind head
- scapulae retracted

Wrist Roller--Extensors (60) 1X6

Captains of Crush Grippers
- Trainer: R:1X5   L:1X5
- #1:   R:1X5   L:2X5
- #1.5:   R:1X5

note: all sets and reps done SLOW & STRICT

Week Three, Day One (Saturday)

Standing 1-Leg Curl (50) 3X15
- Toes Dorsi Flexed (Pulled towards shin)
- Peak Contract

Leg Press (0,50,110) 3X10
- feet straight; close (3.5" apart)
- feet low on platform
- focused on drive through heels ("feel the heels")
- moderate depth, <u>10 rep target</u>
- breathing-style reps 3rd set (3 breaths btwn each rep)

Reverse Hypers-Tilt Forward-With Roller (0+,35+,50+) 3X15,15,25
- Peak Contract
- focused on form, minimizing momentum

Seated 1-leg Hurdler Stretch on Bench 3X each leg
- w/ Jump Stretch Band

Hack Squats (40) 2X12
- Reverse Double Banded
- Heels together, feet at 90 degrees

Standing Thigh/hip flexor stretches 3X each leg

Week Three, Day Two (Sunday)

Incline Press (42) 1X10
    (132,182,222,222)
    4X6,6,6,8
- scapulae retracted
- feet <u>not</u> anchored

Supine db flys (46) 2X20
- Peak Contract
- scapulae retracted

Standing db lateral raises (17.5) 2X15
- brief pause at top of each rep

Side-lying "L" fly (10) 1X20

Dragon Flags 1X15
- Ab board
- 2nd rung up from top

Ab board "Musiek Crunches" 1X25
- vacuum stomach on way down
- legs across bench
- arms across chest

note: performed internal rotator stretches after inclines

Week Three, Day Three (Tuesday)

Seated WIDE Grip Chest Lat Pulldowns
(100,130,130) 3X12,12,15
- Traditional-style bar
- Continuous-style reps

Parallel WIDE Grip KC Rows
(105,150,150) 3X12,15,15+8 SR
- Pause w/ Peak Contract
- SR=Scapular Retractions

Moon Bench db Pullovers (50) 1X20

Seated Toe Raise (100) 3X10
- wide, toes out foot placement
- 1-second pause at top

Standing Tibial Raise 1X50
- heels on mat, toes hanging off
- held onto Incline rack for balance

note: performed internal rotator stretches during rows

note: performed thigh/hip flexor and calf stretches during calves

Week Three, Day Four (Thursday)

Standing EZ "21" Curls (70) 2X"21"
* knurled grip

Seated French Press (60,80) 2X15
* French Curl bar
* no back support

Standing EZ <u>Cable</u> Reverse Curls (40) 1X15
* Lat Machine Low Pulley
* knurled grip
* very slow negatives

Wrist Roller--Flexors (40) 1X5

note: all sets and reps done SLOW & STRICT

Week Four, Day One (Saturday)

Prone Leg Curl (85,105,105) 3X15
- Toes Plantar Flexed (Pointed)
- Peak Contract

Leg Extensions (20,30,30) 3X10,8,8
Banded Walks w/ Bands 1X50
Leg Press-Partials(0,50,90,160) 4X10
- feet straight; close (3.5" apart)
- feet low on platform
- focused on drive through heels ("feel the heels")
- partial depth, 10 rep target
- breathing-style reps 3rd set (3 breaths btwn each rep)

Reverse Hypers-Tilt Forward-With Roller (0+,35+) 2X15,40
- Peak Contract
- focused on form, minimizing momentum

Seated 1-leg Hurdler Stretch on Bench 3X each leg
- w/ Jump Stretch Band

Standing Thigh/hip flexor stretches 3X each leg

Week Four, Day Two (Sunday)

Decline Press (42) 1X10
        (132,182,187,187)
        4X12
           • scapulae retracted
Supine db flys (46) 2X20
   • Peak Contract
   • scapulae retracted

Standing db lateral raises (17.5) 2X15
        • brief pause at top of each rep
Side-lying fly (10) 1X20

Ab Strap Twisting Knee Raise (0) 1X26
      • 13 reps per side
      • Pause w/ Peak Contract
      • slow & controlled w/o any swing
Crunches 1X25
   • feet in air
   • arms across chest
   • supersetted with:
Twisting Alternate Knee-Ins 1X25

Week Four, Day Three (Tuesday)

Parallel WIDE Grip Chins (0,20,20)
>   3X15,12,10
>> • Wide neutral grip attachment

2-Arm Alternate db KC Rows (52.5) 1X15
>> • Pause in top position btwn reps

1-Arm db KC Rows (60) 1X15
>> • Pause w/ Peak Contract

Standing Calf Raises (345) 3X15
- knees locked
- 1-second pause at top

Seated Tibial Raise (32.5) 1X25

note: performed internal rotator stretches during rows

note: performed thigh/hip flexor and calf stretches during calves

note: Chins are tough on the shoulders and are generally only done once every 6-9 months

Week Four, Day Four (Thursday)

Standing Alternate db Curls "Up & Down the Rack"
(20*25*30*35*40*46*40*35*30*25*20)
11X5
- done as one long, continuous set
- Peak Contract every rep

Kneeling on Bench 1-Arm db Kickbacks
(20) 2X12

Wrist Roller--Extensors (60) 1X6

Captains of Crush Grippers
- Trainer: R:1X5   L:1X5
- #1:   R:1X5   L:2X5
- #1.5:   R:1X5

note: all sets and reps done SLOW & STRICT
note: "Up & Down the Rack" is super intense and generally only done once every 3-6 months

Alternative Leg Workout

Standing 1-Leg Curl (50) 3X15
- Toes Dorsi Flexed (Pulled towards shin)
- Peak Contract

Leg Extensions (20) 3X15
Hyperextensions (0) 2X30
Banded Walks w/ Bands 1X50
Hack Squats (40) 3X12
- Reverse Double Banded
- Heels together, feet at 90 degrees

Standing Thigh/hip flexor stretches 3X each leg

note: This workout gets substituted for the scheduled leg day any time I feel like I am not yet fully recovered from the previous leg session.

Chapter 12

Sculpting David

If I trim myself to suit others,
I will soon whittle myself away.
Unknown

I started bodybuilding in 1978 weighing 110 pounds. My most pressing goal at the time was adding muscular bodyweight. With that goal in mind, I ate voraciously, literally turning meal prep into an assembly line production. Breakfast consisted of 3 bowls of cereal, 8 pieces of toast with butter and jelly, a glass of milk and a small glass of grape juice. Altogether, I probably only got 10 grams of protein but prodigious amounts of carbs from that meal! Fortunately, because I was so young and my metabolism was still so high, all of those carbs didn't hurt me any; but the scant amount of protein I ate didn't help me any either. It turns out that only protein supplies the necessary building blocks for adding muscle.

As I mentioned previously, when I began competing, there was no internet yet and books about bodybuilding were few and far between. Books about dieting for competition were nearly non-existent and most of the articles in the muscle magazines were written by, and geared towards, people who were taking steroids. Most of what I learned I learned by asking others who were more accomplished than me and then self-experimenting with their methods.

For my first show, the 1987 Oil City Y.M.C.A. Bodybuilding Championship, I mostly just quit eating. Seriously. I didn't know any better at the time. Then, in 1990, I moved to Canandaigua, NY and joined my first hard core gym, The Fitness Factory. There were always a half dozen or so members getting ready for a competition at any given time. There were bodybuilders, powerlifters, even the gym owner himself had been an Olympic lifter and an alternate for the Olympic Bobsled team. I immersed myself in this great fountain of information. My training and dietary prowess grew exponentially.

It is hard to do justice to this topic in just one chapter. I will state from the outset that this chapter is probably not a very good substitute for a trainer knowledgeable in modern day pre-contest prep. The art of getting ready for show has come a long, long way since my competition days. Nonetheless, I will share with you what worked for me then, what didn't work for me then and what works for me now in my fast-approaching senior years.

My diet regime for my second competition, the 1991 Natural Westmoreland County Championship, was markedly more scientific than anything I had ever attempted up to that point. Instead of just generally focusing on calories, I tracked my macros closely. Protein, carbohydrates and fats make up the macro ingredients that sum together to give you your caloric total, with protein and carbs each contributing four calories per gram and fats contributing nine calories per gram. Specifically, I followed what is sometimes called the "60/30/10 diet" where 60% of my calories were to come from carbohydrate sources, 30% of my calories were to come from protein sources and no more than 10% of my calories were to come from fats. This worked out to be 370 grams of carbs, 150 grams of protein and 20 grams of fats for a caloric total of 2,260. As always, weight loss was to be limited to a maximum of 1.5 to 2 pounds per week to avoid losing muscle. If weight loss started to come too fast, all of the macros were to be boosted accordingly. Meals were spaced evenly throughout each day, eating five to six times.

This was a very difficult regimen to follow. It involved a lot of advance calculation and planning. And, when my weight loss started to accelerate too quickly, it became difficult to eat all of the food necessary to keep the macro ratios intact. Worst of all for me was that, after 6 weeks of following this diet to the letter, I had dropped about 15 pounds but looked exactly like I did before starting the diet, only smaller! My muscular definition had not improved any whatsoever. Clearly, to me, this meant that I was losing muscle, not just fat. My now significantly smaller arms bore this out.

For the remaining 6 weeks of my pre-contest diet, I switched to a radically different tactic. Instead of so diligently tracking all of my macros, I only closely tracked carbs and loosely tracked my protein intake. Specifically, I slashed my carb intake to approximately 70 grams per day, all from simple carb sources. Here's what that looked like: small glass of juice with breakfast (13 grams), 6 ounces of baby food plums mid-morning (30 grams) and eight fudge-covered graham cookies immediately before training to boost my blood sugar levels so I would have enough energy to train (24 grams). Along with this, I ate around 200 grams of protein but, again, I only closely tracked my carbs. The change was nearly immediate and drastic. Suddenly, I was defined. After 6 weeks on this new regimen, I was shredded, albeit smaller than I had hoped to be.

I fine-tuned this diet considerably, and balanced out the health aspects of it much better too, for my next three competitions. I learned to closely track both protein and carb intake; and I learned how to cycle them for best results. Specifically, I kept my protein intake high, between 200-250 grams per day, and I cycled my carb intake such that I ate 55 grams of carbs per day for three successive days followed by a carb-up day of 120 grams on the fourth day. For two of the shows, I was training 3 days on, 1 day off, so the carb-up day always fell on my off days. For the third show, the 1993 N.G.A. Can/Am, I carbed-up every 4th or 5th day, specifically on the day before leg day, regardless of whether it was an off day from training or not. My carb sources all came from complex carbs this time around. Additionally, I purchased, and learned to use, Ketostix to check my ketone levels first thing every morning. Ideally, the strips would start turning dark just prior to my carb-up day and then be clear immediately after. If they got too dark, I would boost my carbs a little to avoid causing any damage to my health. Dieting down in this manner worked amazingly well for me, enabling me to retain most of my hard-earned muscle mass while still coming in shredded.

On the next couple of pages I will share a small sampling from my pre-contest diet journals.

Day 1	P	C
A.M. Ketones "negative"		
9 AM		
1 cup (3 oz,) Oatmeal	15	54
6 egg whites, 3 egg yellows	27	
2:30 PM		
16 oz. chicken breast	74	
8 PM		
10 oz. Porterhouse steak	67	
9 PM		
4 whole eggs	24	
Day 1 Totals	207	54

Day 2	P	C
A.M. Ketones "small"		
6:30 AM		
8 oz. Baked Potato	6	48
6 egg whites, 3 egg yellows	27	
1 medium tomato	1	6
10 AM		
4 egg whites	12	
Noon		
16 oz. chicken breast	74	
4 PM		
4 whole eggs	24	
9 PM		
8 oz. ground beef	53	
2 whole eggs	12	
Day 2 Totals	209	54

Day 3	P	C
A.M. Ketones "small"		
6:30 AM		
1 cup (3 oz.) Oatmeal	15	54
6 egg whites, 3 egg yellows	27	
10 AM		
4 egg whites, 2 egg yellows	18	
Noon		
16 oz. chicken breast	74	
4 PM		
4 egg whites, 2 egg yellows	18	
9:40 PM		
8 oz. ground beef	53	
Day 3 Totals	205	54

Day 4	P	C
A.M. Ketones "medium"		
6:30 AM		
8 oz. Baked Potato	6	48
6 egg whites, 3 egg yellows	27	
1 medium tomato	1	6
10 AM		
5 oz. brown rice	3	41
Noon		
16 oz. chicken breast	74	
4 PM		
4 whole eggs	24	
9 PM		
4 oz. yellow corn w/ butter	4	25
9 oz. ground beef	61	
Day 4 Totals	200	120

As I have gotten older, my metabolism has slowed down considerably. When I was 25 years old, about a year before I really started competing regularly, I noticed that I had gained a little fat around my middle. So, I went out and purchased a rebounder, one of those mini trampolines that you run on. I ran on it for a half an hour every day for one week and dropped 10 pounds and reduced my waist size by 1.5 inches. Then, when I was 35 years old, I noticed that I had gotten considerably fatter than before around my middle. So, I got my rebounder back out and ran on it every day for half an hour for an entire year and I never lost one pound!

Nowadays, at 55 years of age, I focus more on portion control, rarely partaking of second helpings, eating salads as my lunch 3-4X per week and still getting ample amounts of protein, mostly through my home concocted protein drink recipe.

Jon's Protein Drinks	
2 cups (16 oz.) 2% milk	16g
1/3 cup Vanilla Yogurt	3-6g
1 cup Powdered Milk	34g
Total	53-56g

If I notice my weight starting to increase when I don't want it to, I slightly reduce my carb intake, but generally not my protein intake which I now keep around 150-200 grams a day on training days and 100 grams on non-training days.

I have never been a big fan of taking large amounts of supplements. Yes, in 42 years of training, I have certainly tried my fair share. But, most of them just don't work. Wonder products come and go like the changing of the seasons. Any product that gets marketed as "almost as good as steroids" or "so powerful it should be illegal" is garbage; snake oil salesman peddling their wares. The only products out there that truly are as good as steroids are steroids and those are illegal, in most instances, and come with a whole host of undesirable side-effects.

I do like a good protein powder. By "good" I mean one that is a quality protein source without having a bunch of unnecessary and questionable added ingredients mixed in. If you look, you can find them. But, as I stated previously, I mostly make my own now. Other than that, the only supplements I take on a regular basis are a good multi-mineral, because minerals are easily depleted through sweat when training, a B-Complex and Vitamin D. I prefer multi-minerals to taking individual minerals because they are more readily absorbed when they are in the proper balanced ratios to one another. If I am feeling a little under the weather, I will add some powdered Vitamin C into the mix as well. I steer clear of energy drinks and pre-workout mixes. All of that caffeine can be hard on your system.

As for cardio, when I was competing, I would get up first thing in the morning and ride a stationary bike with zero tension for 30-60 minutes. The reason for setting the tension at zero was because I already had a workout program for my legs; this was just for stoking my metabolism. I have a Schwinn Airdyne now, but I am very cautious about how hard I push myself on it because, again, it's not how much training you can do, it's how much training you can recover from. I have found that I can easily overdo myself with this particular bike. My preferred method of cardio nowadays is boxing cardio, hitting the speed bag and the heavy bag for several 3-minute rounds with only a 30 second break between rounds.

Chapter 13

Mousetraps

If you build a better mousetrap,
the world will beat a path to your door.
Unknown

A lot of controversy surrounds the above quote, concerning its origin, with various "authorities" crediting it to Ralph Waldo Emerson, Elbert Hubbard, Sarah S. B. Yule, John R. Paxton and Orison Swett Marden. Regardless of its origin, however, it has come to be accepted as fact by most. If you repeat a fairy tale often enough, and with enough *conviction*, it starts to look and feel like an apparent truth to the masses, even though it is still false. Such is the case with this quote.

In the early 1900s, electric trolley cars were plentiful in the big cities. They were comfortable, quiet, dependable and relatively mild in terms of any negative environmental impact. Then, in the 1930s, the switch from rail-to-rubber began as tire and oil conglomerates touted the merits of buses: they were faster, had a greater reach and were promoted heavily as being more modern and stylish. They were also, at least initially, uncomfortable, noisy, more prone to breakdown and veritable titans at spewing carbon monoxide into the atmosphere. Despite these shortcomings, they quickly supplanted their rivals.

Sadly, stories like these are not the exception. During the 1930s, B.J. Palmer, son of the man who discovered Chiropractic, and the driving force behind the profession for over 60 years, set up his own research facility in Davenport, Iowa. One of his many inventions, and certainly the most significant one was a device he named the electro-encephalo-neuro-men-timp-o-graph, a device which consisted of numerous, large cabinets filled with test tubes, enough to completely fill a large room, and used to measure transmission of "mental impulse" between the brain and the body, before and after adjustment. Through his research facility, he was able to demonstrate significant reductions in mental impulse conduction at the level of the spine most in need of a Chiropractic adjustment; and, by precisely adjusting patients at said level, countless scores of otherwise hopeless patients regained their health. To this day, nobody knows, for sure, what he was even measuring! All that remains today of his invention are a couple of cabinets, now housed in a museum.

There is no beaten path. I suspect that many a "better mousetrap" has been lost to the sands of time, aided and abetted by ignorance, greed, poor marketing and unfortunate timing.

Back in 2000, while following an intense squat program, several previously injured discs in my back finished letting go, resulting in a condition known as foot drop, and necessitating many months of chiropractic care and rehabilitative exercises before regaining most of the function and sensation in my right foot. Subsequent to this, two exercises I had previously tolerated well, and relied heavily upon, were now out: barbell bent-over rows and good mornings. Even using nothing heavier than an empty 45 pound Olympic bar for either of these exercises was enough to make my foot start to tingle again. Thus began the search for comparable replacements.

Supported row benches are plentiful, yet most, perhaps all, rely upon the same basic design: a long-axis support board to lay prone on and some lever or specialized bar to add weight to. Barbell rows have always been one of my favorite exercises, and one my body has always responded well to. However, with every bench I tried, the support board itself, pressing against my abdomen, made breathing difficult and uncomfortable, if not impossible. Most of the bars had to travel a greatly reduced path of motion, as well, due to the presence of the board. There are some very interesting machine rows on the market as well, but, for me, the feel was never quite the same.

Then, one day, while glancing at one of the specialized Chiropractic tables in my office, one known as a Gonstead Knee-Chest Table, the idea thought flashed into my head. What if there was a row bench, configured similar to this particular Chiropractic table, where I could kneel in position, with my chest and head supported similarly, but my abdomen completely unencumbered? This would facilitate taking all of the stress off of my lower back while allowing for complete range of motion with a regular barbell and freedom to breathe too. And so, the Knee Chest Row Bench was born. The adrenaline rush that accompanied this thought flash is hard to put into words. I thought I had found my very own "better mousetrap."

So sure was I of this new concept, that I immediately set about filing for a patent, before even making my first prototype. Patents are very expensive to file for and take a considerable amount of time to establish. During this time, I started contacting every weight equipment manufacturer, muscle-oriented magazine publisher and pro-level athlete in any way connected to the sport. Most did not reply at all; and, with two exceptions, the ones that did reply were all negative. Powerlifting USA magazine ran a free promo for me. Robert Kennedy, owner of the MuscleMag International publishing empire in Toronto, was the other.

Mr. Kennedy REALLY liked the concept and replied back, "you really have to make a prototype," offering to test it for me in their corporate headquarters gym. This is the closest I ever came to actually getting this bench into the marketplace.

First, I had a prototype made for myself, so I could test it in relation to my lower back issues. It worked exceptionally well, but needed a few more tweaks before sending it to Canada. For one thing, a foot anchor needed to be added to prevent sliding off the bench when the weights got heavy. The man who was manufacturing my prototypes was located several states away and supplied me with numerous pieces for my home gym over the years. I sent him the list of modifications and paid him additional to then send it directly to Mr. Kennedy.

Unfortunately for me, the bench that was sent to Canada, the 2nd bench made for me by this manufacturer, was completely unusable because the barbell support racks were placed directly in line with the headpiece center post, making it impossible to even put a barbell on it. After this, Mr. Kennedy was kind enough to gift me with a signed, 1st edition of MuscleMag International, for my trouble, when I showed up to retrieve my bench. But, other than also giving me a free promo in his magazine as well, he asked that I not send him another bench.

Ultimately, after spending more than $10,000 and working at it for four years, the Knee Chest Row Bench was successfully patented, receiving U.S. Patent #7,128,701. [See Appendix A] Seven years later, having only ever sold two benches, and in the throes of other financial trouble, I had to let the patent expire.

In spite of all this, the Knee Chest Row Bench was, and is, my better mousetrap. It has allowed me to continue doing heavy barbell rows for the past 17 years. Subsequent modifications, allowed for the headpiece to be used in both kneeling, as well as, standing configurations. Further, it has allowed for the introduction of several unique exercises into my training program, including 2-Arm Alternate Dumbbell Rows and Barbell Spider Curls too.

As a gift to you the reader, I have included, as an Appendix to this book, the official CAD drawings that were created for this bench so you too can make your own if you so desire. [See Appendix B] For those so inclined, the unit can be made more sanitary, for use in large-scale, commercial gym applications, through the addition of a holder for a roll of Chiropractic headrest paper.

About the Author

I have always loved bodybuilding, its Zen nature, the solo pursuit of excellence. It has been the one constant in my life through good times and bad times alike.

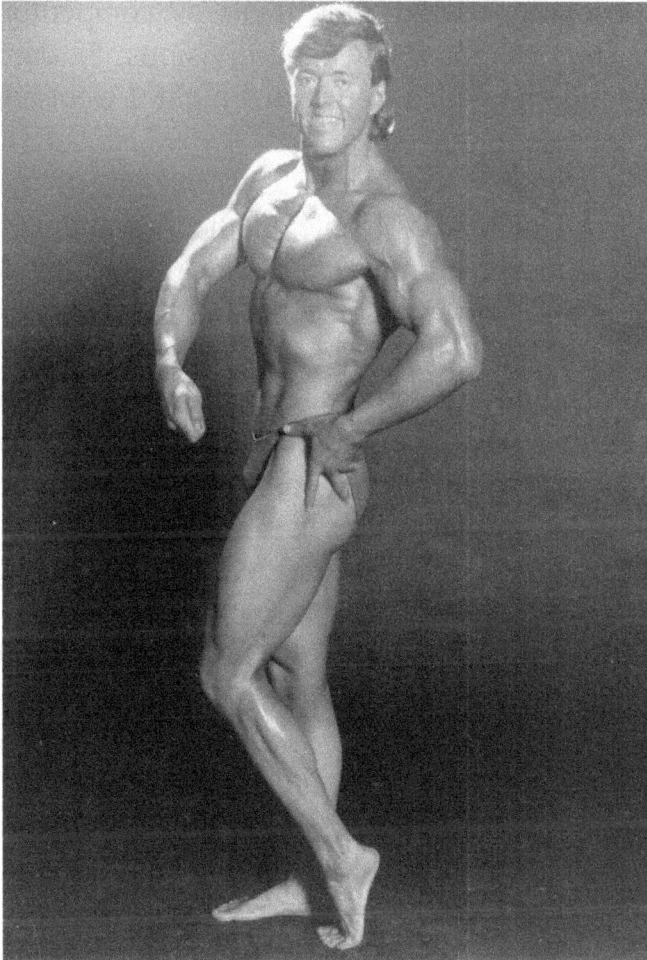

My competitive career in bodybuilding moved between extremes. The 1991 A.N.B.C. Natural Westmoreland Bodybuilding Classic was my first really big show and my biggest loss as well. The show was structured such that the top four competitors in each class got a trophy; anyone who didn't earn a trophy that day was to be given a consolation medal. Out of the 59 competitors in the various weight classes and divisions, 58 competitors went home with a trophy that night. I went home with a consolation medal.

Undaunted, I entered the first annual N.G.A. Can/Am six months later. The novice division was huge and split into short and tall classes, whereas the open division was split between short, medium and tall. Nobody was measured the day of the show; they went by what the competitors had self-reported on their entry paperwork. I am 5'8", at best. But, I have an older brother who is 6'4" and I had always thought I would end up taller too; I didn't. Anyways, on my entry paperwork for this particular show, I was wishful thinking and listed my height as 5' 8 1/2". I had no way of predicting where the cut-offs would be for each height class, which turned out to be up to 5'8" for the short class and everyone over 5'8" for the tall class. I was the shortest "tall" competitor in the novice tall class that day out of 17 contestants.

Nonetheless, I held my own. Only the top three were placed but, had they placed a fourth, it would have been between myself and one other competitor who the judges kept comparing me to. In the open division, they also only placed the top three, or so I thought. Several months later, I read the contest results in Natural Physique magazine and saw that I had actually been awarded 4th place in the open division. Immediately after the show, I approached the judges, as I always did after competition, to ask for feedback on how I could do better. The first judge I approached told me, "I don't even remember who you are; there were so many competitors!" The second judge I approached was far kinder and more compassionate. He actually told me, "I don't know why you didn't place. I had you in 2nd on my score card," which he retrieved and gave to me. He followed up by mailing me a letter where he reiterated that he felt I should have placed 2nd that day. I cannot begin to tell you how much that meant to me. I still have his letter, framed on my wall.

The N.G.A. Buffalo Classic was a major turning point for me. I won 1st place in the open middleweight division and, in doing so, defeated two competitors whom I had faced at the Can/Am: the competitor whom I had been compared to so rigorously in the novice division, tall class and the competitor who had won 2nd place in the open division, medium class, where one judge in particular felt I had been overlooked.

In reality, the only one I was ever competing against was myself. There's no way to predict who will show up at any given show and there is always somebody better than you out there. My focus was always on improving my own level of condition from show-to-show, regardless of how high or low my final placement might be. You have to learn to believe in yourself, even when nobody else does.

I was training at State Street Gym in Iowa one day when one of the local gym rats came over to give me a hard time while I was practicing my posing between sets. I was completely covered, wearing a rag top and baggies, so it wasn't like I was showing off my physique or anything like that. I was just going about my training. I had just recently moved to Iowa from New York to attend Chiropractic school. I had also just taken 2nd place at the second annual Can/Am a couple of months before. "You're not big enough to be posing," he told me. "I've got a bunch of trophies on my dresser at home that says I am!" I replied.

Bodybuilding Resume

Bodybuilding – since 12/78

Competitions:
- 1987 Oil City YMCA Bodybuilding Championship – 4th Place (July 1987)
- 1991 A.N.B.C. Natural Westmoreland Bodybuilding Classic (Sept. 1991)
- 1992 N.G.A. Can/Am Bodybuilding Championship – 4th Place (May 1992)
- 1992 N.G.A. Natural Buffalo Classic – 1st Place (November 1992)
- 1993 N.G.A. Can/Am Bodybuilding Championship – 2nd Place (May 1993)
- 2001 N.G.A. Can/Am Bodybuilding Championship – withdrew (April 2001)
- 2005 N.G.A. Olympus – 5th place (October 2005)

Judge:
- 2001 N.G.A. Olympus
- 2002 N.G.A. Can/Am Bodybuilding Championship
- 2002 N.G.A. Olympus
- 2003 N.G.A. Can/Am Bodybuilding Championship
- 2003 N.G.A. Olympus

- **2004 N.G.A. Can/Am Bodybuilding Championship**
- **2007 N.G.A. Can/Am Bodybuilding Championship**
- **2008 N.G.A. Can/Am Bodybuilding Championship**
- **2010 N.G.A. Can/Am Bodybuilding Championship**
- **2011 N.M.A. Can/Am Bodybuilding Championship**
- **2012 N.M.A. Olympus**
- **2013 N.M.A. Can/Am Bodybuilding Championship**
- **2013 N.M.A. Great Lakes Championship**
- **2013 N.M.A. Olympus**
- **2014 N.M.A. Great Lakes Championship**
- **2014 N.M.A. Can/Am Bodybuilding Championship**

Promoter:
- **2011 N.M.A. The Reach for the Ring**

The Reach for the Ring

Connecting with the Author

Websites:
www.AlwaysBelieveInYourDreams.com
www.TheReachForTheRing.com
[under construction]

Social Media:

Instagram:
@hearton4lifting
@jon.m.ketcham

Facebook:
Jon M. Ketcham

LinkedIn:
jon m ketcham

YouTube Channel:
Jon Ketcham

Twitter:
@jon_m_ketcham

Pinterest:
jon m ketcham

Other Books by jon m ketcham

Ask Me Who I Was - *audacious brain farts on life, death and immortality*

The Golden Role - *Just Be Nice!*

The "Zero's Journey" - *A Modern-day Survival Guide to Weathering Accidental Enlightenment*

iContractor1 - *Constructing Your Perfect Life by Remodeling YOU from the Inside-Out!*

Appendix A

US007128701B1

(12) **United States Patent**　　　(10) **Patent No.:**　　**US 7,128,701 B1**
Ketcham　　　　　　　　　　　(45) **Date of Patent:**　　Oct. 31, 2006

(54) **KNEE-CHEST ROWING BENCH**

(76) Inventor: **Jon M. Ketcham**, 947 C St.,
Meadville, PA (US) 16335

(*) Notice: Subject to any disclaimer, the term of this
patent is extended or adjusted under 35
U.S.C. 154(b) by 0 days.

(21) Appl. No.: **10/455,841**

(22) Filed: **Jun. 6, 2003**

(51) Int. Cl.
A63B 26/00 (2006.01)
(52) U.S. Cl. 482/142; 482/148
(58) Field of Classification Search 482/142,
482/148, 907, 91; D21/676, 686, 690, 622
See application file for complete search history.

(56) **References Cited**

U.S. PATENT DOCUMENTS

4,625,962 A	*	12/1986	Street	.... 482/116
5,169,363 A	*	12/1992	Campanaro et al.	.... 482/96
5,971,485 A	*	10/1999	Clark	.... 297/423.12
6,065,808 A	*	5/2000	Tinsley	.... 297/423.11
6,149,556 A	*	11/2000	Jordan	.... 482/104
6,543,853 B1	*	4/2003	Splane, Jr.	.... 297/423.12
6,726,607 B1	*	4/2004	Ihli	.... 482/127
2002/0002104 A1	*	1/2002	Panatta	.... 482/93
2004/0070253 A1	*	4/2004	Murphy et al.	.... 297/423.11

* cited by examiner

Primary Examiner—Lori Amerson
(74) *Attorney, Agent, or Firm*—Jonathan M. D'Silva;
MacDonald, Illig, Jones & Britton LLP

(57) **ABSTRACT**

A kneeling bench and a head rest with a face opening afford
a user a way to be comfortably situated in a face down
position to perform rowing motions with free weights or
weight stacks. The lateral distance between the two bench
elements can be adjusted as can the vertical distance to
accommodate different sized users. In addition the angle of
the head rest is adjustable between angles of 25° and 35°
from the horizontal.

21 Claims, 1 Drawing Sheet

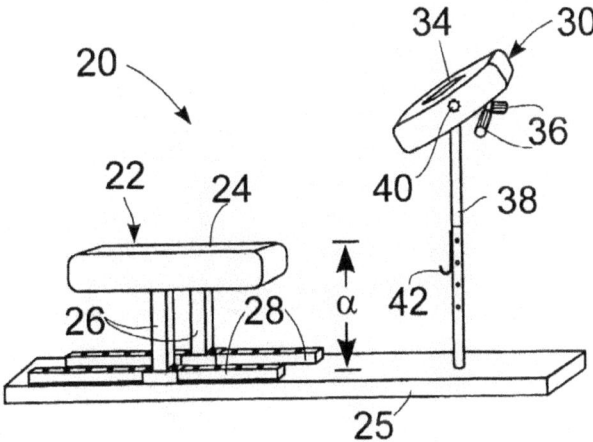

The Reach for the Ring

Appendix A

U.S. Patent   Oct. 31, 2006   US 7,128,701 B1

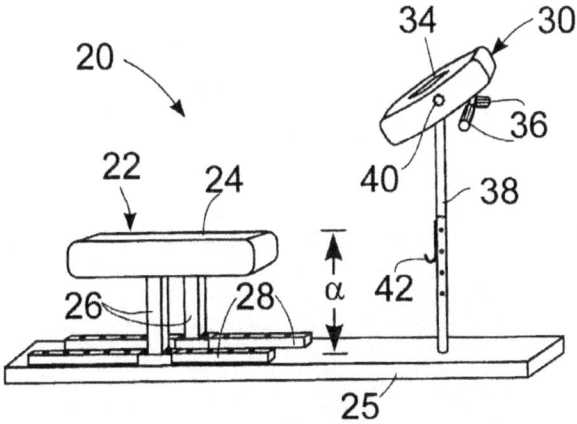

Fig. 1

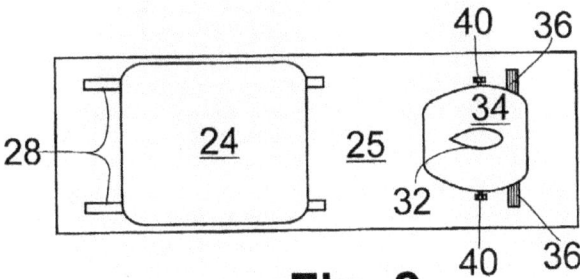

Fig. 2

The Reach for the Ring

Appendix A

US 7,128,701 B1

1

KNEE-CHEST ROWING BENCH

This invention was disclosed in Disclosure Document No. 514,906 filed Jul. 15, 2002.

BACKGROUND AND SUMMARY OF THE INVENTION

The present invention is directed to the field of exercise devices. More particularly, the present invention is directed to a bench which supports the user's weight via a kneeling bench and a headrest leaving a zone from the mid-sternum to the knees open to permit a rowing arm motion.

The exercise equipment industry has mushroomed in the last 10 years. In the same time period, health clubs have grown in numbers and membership. The equipment used in health clubs is typically complex and expensive. Home gymnasiums, while providing numerous exercise options, are often complicated and difficult to use. Our lives, already complicated by work and family, cry out for simplicity to provide relief in the area of exercise.

The knee-chest rowing bench of the present invention provides a simplicity that is elegant, providing a face-downward support that comfortably supports the user's weight while permitting a significant range of motion for both arms simultaneously or, each arm individually. The user can use the bench with free weights such as barbells and dumbbells or with weight stacks employing cables and pulleys. The bench of the present invention is designed to provide the benefits of the barbell bent over rowing without the risks. Bent over rows are very effective exercise for the upper back but a dangerously strenuous exercise for the lower back.

Other attempts at providing a supported-type of bent-over row unit have typically relied on a long-axis support (i.e., a padded board) which runs continuously from episternal notch down to the umbilicus (navel) or lower. However, this type of support creates two problems: first, it interferes with breathing due to compressing the rib cage and abdomen against the board. Second, the support board acts as an obstacle or barrier since, in this exercise, the barbell is meant to be pulled into a zone ranging from just inferior to the nipple line (imaginary horizontal line connecting both nipples) down to the umbilicus. In this instance, the support board acts to decrease the effective range of motion (ROM).

One arm dumbbell rows are sometimes performed as a substitute for barbell bent-over rows. However, this exercise is considered secondary, at best, in terms of effectiveness. Furthermore, the stabilizing arm, which is kept straight, tends to bear an increased amount of stress to the shoulder and rotator cuff musculature.

The knee-chest rowing bench of the present invention includes plural support surfaces including a kneeling platform at a first level for supporting a majority of the user's body weight in a kneeling position at a height in the range from one foot to two feet from a floor; a headrest for at a second level above said first level for supporting the user's head in a face down orientation; the plural support surfaces supporting the user's full weight leaving unencumbered a zone at least between the user's mid-sternum and navel to facilitate arm motion and breathing at a height sufficient to permit the user's arms to swing in a fully extended position without contacting the floor.

The exercise bench preferably has means to adjust both the horizontal and vertical distances between the headrest and the kneeling bench, in order to comfortably accommodate individual body sizes and shapes. The headrest prefer-

2

ably has an opening in its upper supporting surface to comfortably accommodate the user's face. The angularity of the headrest is preferably adjustable between a range of 25° and 35°, again, in order to accommodate personal preference and afford maximum comfort. A pair of, preferably, vertically oriented handles are positioned either side of the headrest to provide the user balance while doing rowing exercises with the opposite hand.

The knee-chest rowing bench of the present invention is geared to the serious weight trainee, be it a school athlete, body builder, fitness enthusiast or dedicated home trainee.

Various other features, advantages and characteristics of the present invention will become apparent to one of ordinary skill in the art after a reading of the following specification.

BRIEF DESCRIPTION OF THE DRAWINGS

The preferred embodiment(s) of the present invention is/are described in conjunction with the associated drawings in which like features are indicated with like reference numerals and in which

FIG. 1 is a side view of a first embodiment of the exercise bench of the present invention; and

FIG. 2 is a top view of the first embodiment.

DETAILED DESCRIPTION OF PREFERRED EMBODIMENT(S)

A first embodiment of the knee-chest rowing bench of the present invention is depicted in FIGS. 1 and 2 generally at 20. Exercise bench 20 of the present invention has two main components: kneeling bench 22 and head rest 30. Kneeling bench 20 supports the majority of the user's body weight in a kneeling position on support pad 24 via legs 26 a distance α from the nearest floor, in this case, support pallet 25. The distance α is preferably in the range of between one foot and two feet from the floor with α most preferably being 18". This distance, coupled with the upward body slant afforded by the position of head rest 30, will enable the user to freely swing her/his arm beneath her/him without contacting the floor 25. While knee-chest rowing bench 20 is shown anchored to a support pallet, in a health club environment, elements 22 and 30 could obviously be mounted directly to the floor. Legs 26 are shown mounted on tracks 28 to permit toward and away movement relative to the head rest 30. This enables bench 20 to comfortably accommodate different sized body frames.

Head rest 30 has a face opening 32 to permit the user to support her/his head on the pillow 34 without smashing her/his nose. This provides head/neck support in neutral position without any rotation or extension of the cervical spine. In addition, opening 32 will permit some visibility of the hand motion during the exercise. It is contemplated that if bench 20 is employed for home use, the user will most typically use hand weights to swing to-and-fro in a sweeping motion beneath her/his suspended frame. Both arms can be swung simultaneously, while using a barbell or pair of dumbbells. By grasping handle 36 on the offside for balance while alternately working the arm/shoulder muscles of first the left side and then the right, dumbbell rows could also be performed one arm at a time. While the handles 36 have been shown as extending laterally, for ease of depiction, they will more preferably, have a vertically extending, graspable portion to enhance stability of the user. A pair of racks 42 (one shown) are positioned on the front of the support stand 38 to accommodate a barbell (not shown). It will be under-

The Reach for the Ring

Appendix A

US 7,128,701 B1

3

stood that the racks 42 could be free standing supporting the barbell in a similar position. The user may grasp the barbell with both hands and pull it upwardly to contact her/his chest in a rowing motion. Since the knee-chest rowing bench of the present invention leaves the user's torso unencumbered, this rowing exercise, as well as a number of others, is facilitated.

Two additional adjustments are provided; first, the height of support stand 38 can be adjusted vertically, again, to accommodate various builds of users. The adjustment is shown as a pin in aligned holes of telescoping tubes, although it will be appreciated that other adjustment means could be used. Second, the tilt angle of the head rest 30 can be adjusted, preferably within a range of 25° and 35° from horizontal, by loosening then tightening knurled knobs 40 to lock head rest 30 at the desired angular position, although it will be appreciated that other adjustment means could be used.

By adjusting the distance between the kneeling bench 22 and head rest 30, the height of head rest 30 and the angle of pillow 34, the exercise bench 20 of the present invention can be configured to comfortably accommodate any user. The handles 36 afford a means of balance for the offhand side while the user uses free weights or weight stacks to exercise the opposite arm/shoulder muscle group. The knee-chest rowing bench 20 of the present invention provides a simple, effective bench permitting upper body exercises, particularly barbell bent-over rows, 2-arm dumbbell rows, and 1-arm dumbbell rows. These exercises can be performed by a user who is comfortably positioned without a) compromising lower back or shoulder safety (as free standing versions do) and b) compromising breathing and range of motion (as supported versions do).

Various changes, alternatives and modifications will become apparent to one of ordinary skill in the art following a reading of the foregoing specification. It is intended that any such changes, alternatives and modifications as fall within the scope of the appended claims be considered part of the present invention.

I claim:

1. An exercise bench with plural support surfaces for supporting a user for upper body exercise, said plural support surfaces comprising:

  (a) a kneeling platform at a first level for supporting a majority of the user's body weight in a kneeling position at a height in the range from one foot to two feet from a floor;

  (b) a headrest at a second level spaced by a first vertical distance above said first level and by a second horizontal distance for supporting the user's head in a face down orientation, said headrest including an opening in said headrest sized to comfortably accommodate a user's face;

said plural support surfaces being spaced horizontally and vertically to support the user's full weight in a face down, kneeling position, said weight being distributed between the user's knees and portions of her/his face leaving unencumbered and unsupported a zone at least between the user's mid-sternum and navel to facilitate arm motion and breathing at a height sufficient to permit the user's arms to swing in a fully extended position without contacting the floor.

2. The exercise bench of claim 1 wherein said plural support surfaces are spaced horizontally and vertically to provide a zone unencumbered and unsupported by said support surfaces extending at least between the user's mid-sternum and the user's knees.

4

3. The exercise bench of claim 1 further comprising means for adjusting said second horizontal distance between said kneeling platform and said headrest.

4. The exercise bench of claim 1 further comprising means for adjusting said second level vertically to alter said first vertical distance above said first level of said kneeling platform to accommodate a user's body size and provide maximum comfort.

5. The exercise bench of claim 1 wherein said opening is provided by a space formed between two portions of a split headrest.

6. The exercise bench of claim 1 further comprising means to position said headrest at an angle to horizontal in a range between 25° and 35°.

7. The exercise bench of claim 6 wherein said angle to the horizontal is most preferably 30°.

8. The exercise bench of claim 6 further comprising means for adjusting said headrest throughout said range.

9. The exercise bench of claim 1 further comprising a pair of handles positioned on either side of said headrest to facilitate one-armed exercises by grasping an off-sided handle with the user's opposing hand.

10. The exercise bench of claim 1 further comprising support rack means for suspending a barbell therefrom.

11. The exercise bench of claim 3 wherein said means for adjusting said second horizontal distance comprises rail means upon which one of said plural support surfaces slide in a horizontal direction.

12. An exercise bench with plural support surfaces for supporting a user for upper body exercise, said plural support surfaces comprising:

  a first support surface comprising a kneeling platform at a first level at a height in the range from one foot to two feet from a floor;

  a second support surface comprising a headrest at a second level, said second support surface including an opening in said headrest sized to accommodate a user's face; and

  said second level spaced at a vertical distance above said first level and a horizontal distance from said first level such that said first support surface supports a majority of the user's body weight in a kneeling position and said second support surface supports the user's upper body in a face down orientation by contacting the user's body at a position on the user's body that includes at least the user's mid-sternum and above, said first and second support surfaces spaced to leave unencumbered and unsupported a zone at least between the first and second support surfaces to permit the user to make rowing arm motions beneath the user's suspended frame using a barbell, a dumbbell, or a pair of dumbbells.

13. The exercise bench of claim 12 further comprising a vertical adjuster for adjusting said vertical distance between said first support surface and said second support surface.

14. The exercise bench of claim 12 further comprising a horizontal adjuster for adjusting said horizontal distance between said first support surface and said second support surface.

15. The exercise bench of claim 12 further comprising a horizontal adjuster for adjusting said horizontal distance between said first support surface and said second support surface wherein said horizontal adjuster comprises a rail upon which one of said plural support surfaces can slide in a horizontal direction.

The Reach for the Ring

Appendix A

US 7,128,701 B1

5

16. The exercise bench of claim 12 wherein said opening is provided by a space formed between two portions of a split headrest.

17. The exercise bench or claim 12 further comprising means to position said second support surface at an angle to horizontal in a range between about 25° and about 35°.

18. The exercise bench of claim 12 wherein said second support surface is at an angle to the horizontal of about 30°.

19. The exercise bench of claim 12 further comprising a pair of handles positioned under said second support surface on either side of said second support surface.

20. The exercise bench of claim 12 further comprising support rack means for suspending a barbell therefrom.

21. An exercise bench with plural support surfaces for supporting a user for upper body exercise, said plural support surfaces comprising:

a first support surface comprising a kneeling platform at a first level at a height in the range from one foot to two feet from a floor;

a second support surface comprising a headrest at a second level, said second support surface including an opening in said headrest sized to accommodate a user's face;

said second level spaced at a vertical distance above said first level and a horizontal distance from said first level such that said first support surface supports a majority

6

of the user's body weight in a kneeling position and said second support surface supports the user's upper body in a face down orientation by contacting the user's body at a position on the user's body that includes at least the user's mid-sternum and above, said first and second support surfaces spaced to leave unencumbered and unsupported a zone at least between the first and second support surfaces to permit the user to make rowing arm motions beneath the user's suspended frame using a barbell, a dumbbell, or a pair of dumbbells;

a vertical adjuster for adjusting said vertical distance between said first support surface and said second support surface;

a horizontal adjuster for adjusting said horizontal distance between said first support surface and said second support surface;

means to position said second support surface at an angle to horizontal in a range between about 25° and about 35°;

a pair of handles positioned under said second support surface on either side of said second support surface; and

support rack means for suspending a barbell therefrom.

* * * * *

The Reach for the Ring

Appendix B - CAD Drawings

The Reach for the Ring

The Reach for the Ring

Appendix B - CAD Drawings

177

Appendix B - CAD Drawings

The Reach for the Ring

Appendix B - CAD Drawings

The Reach for the Ring

The Reach for the Ring

Appendix B - CAD Drawings

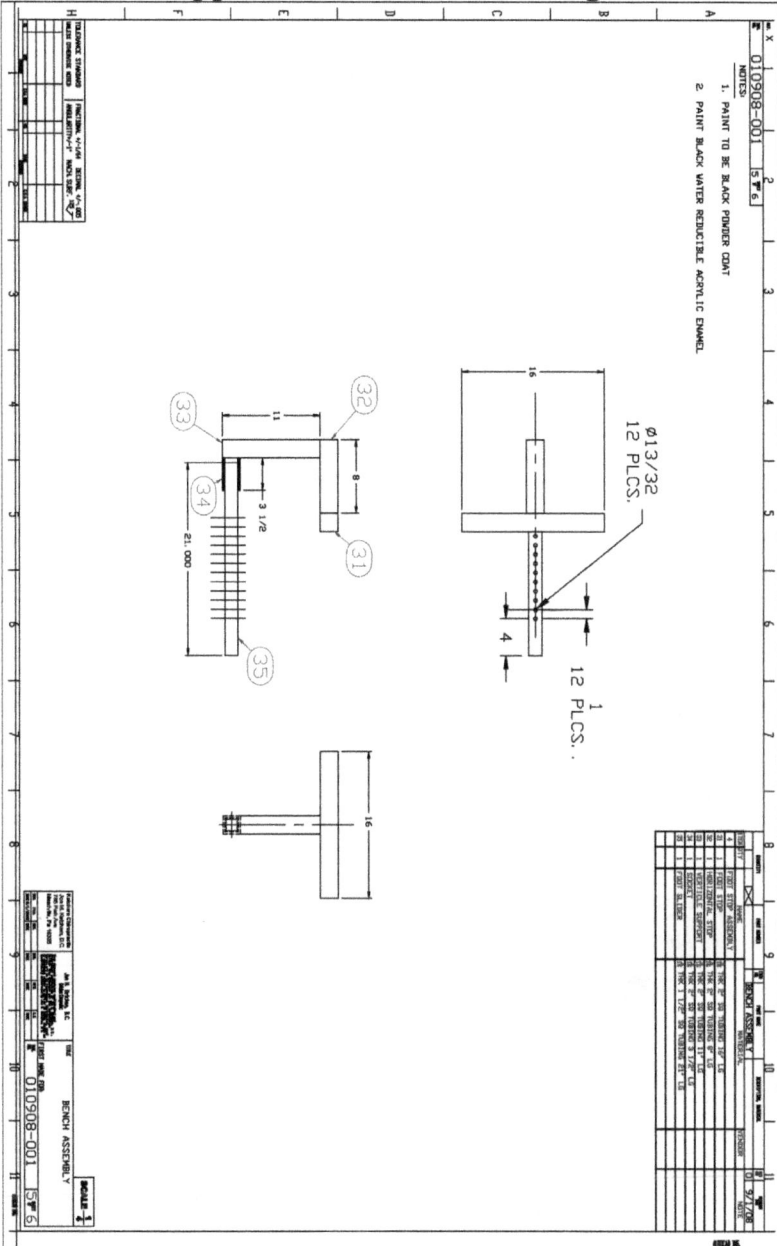

183

The Reach for the Ring

Appendix B - CAD Drawings

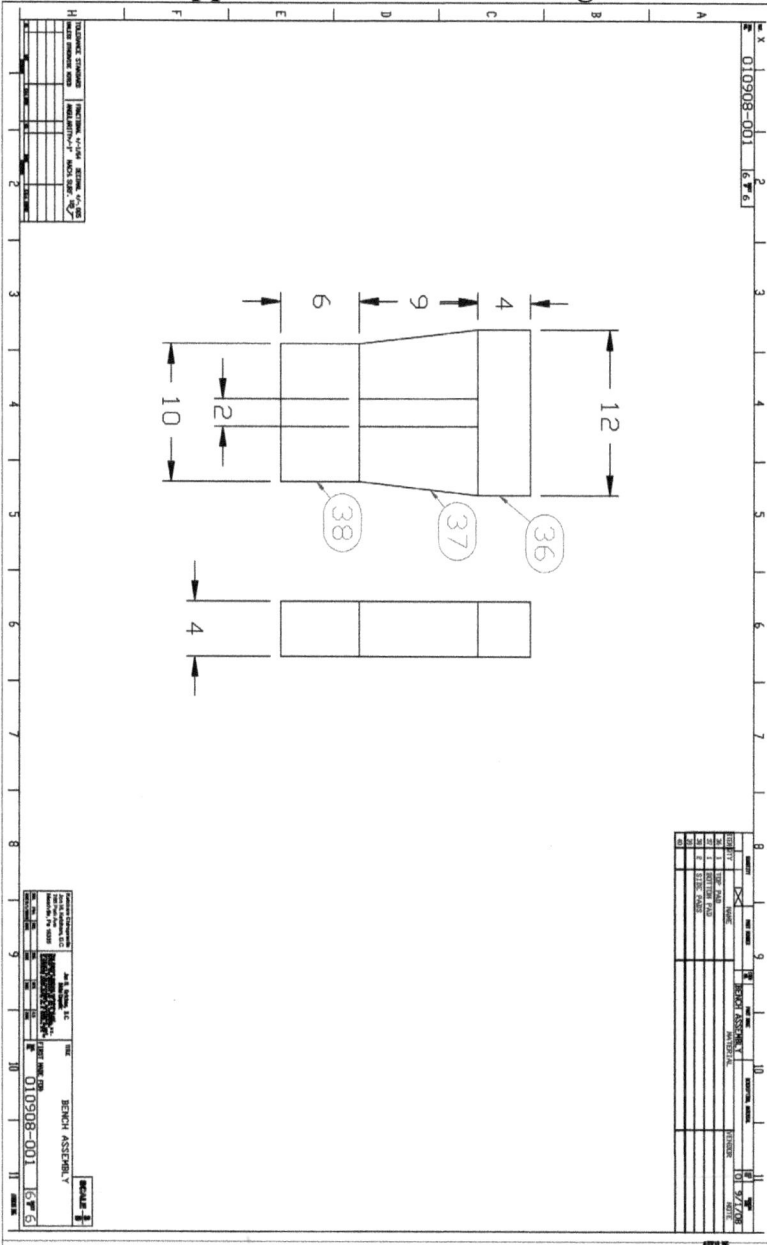

Appendix C

KC Row Bench Prototype

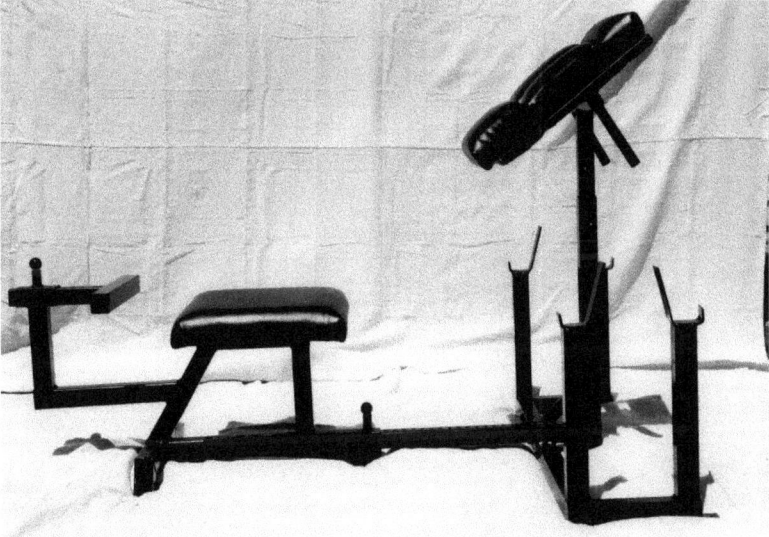

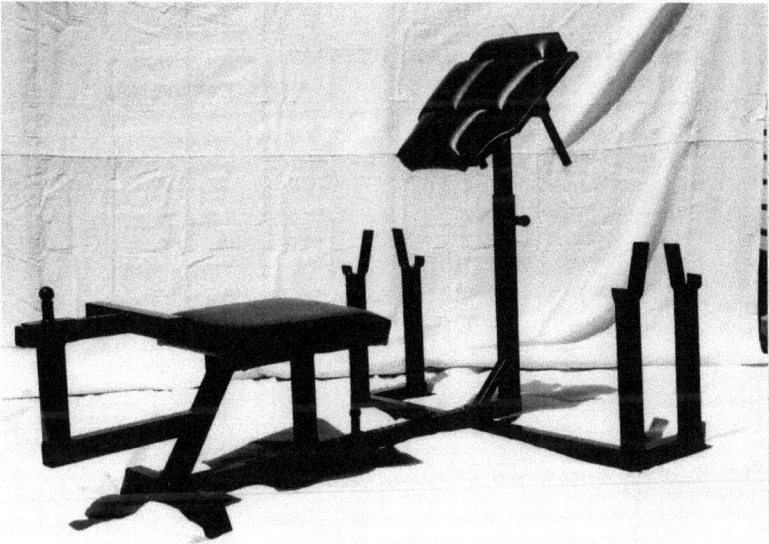

The Reach for the Ring

Appendix C

KC Row Bench Prototype

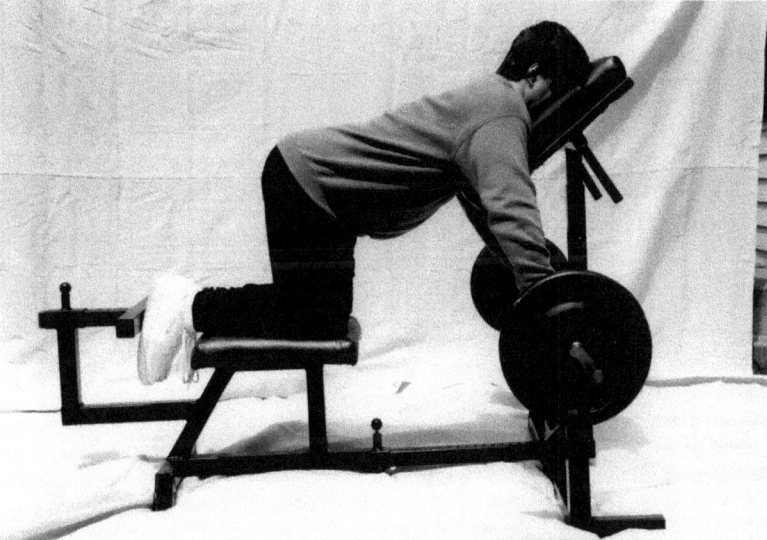

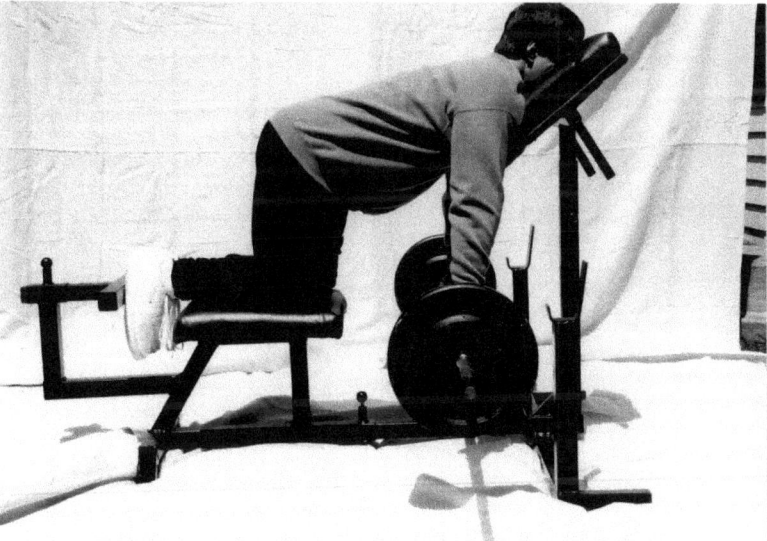

The Reach for the Ring

Appendix C

KC Row Bench Prototype

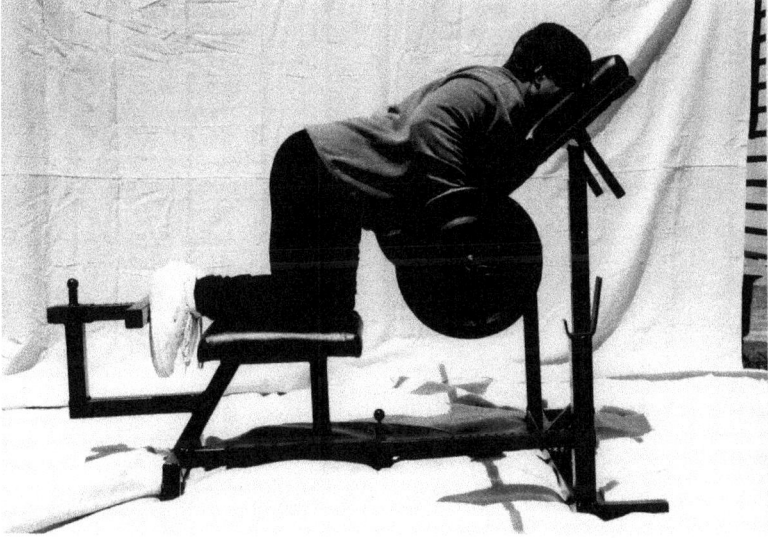

The Reach for the Ring

Appendix C

KC Row Bench Prototype

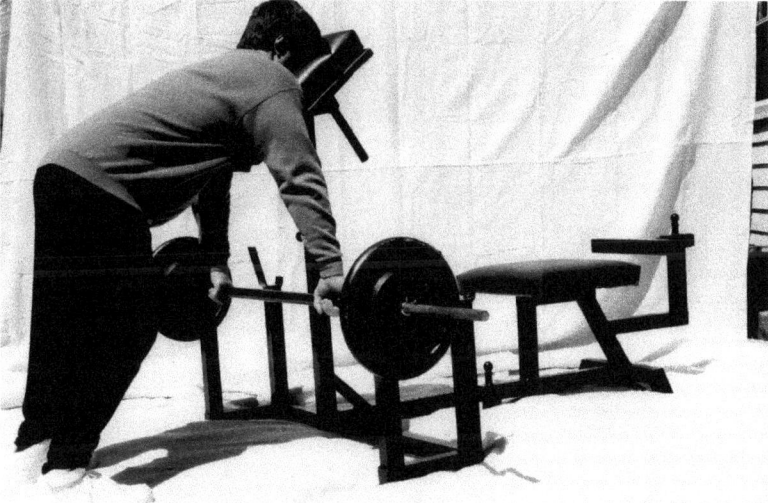

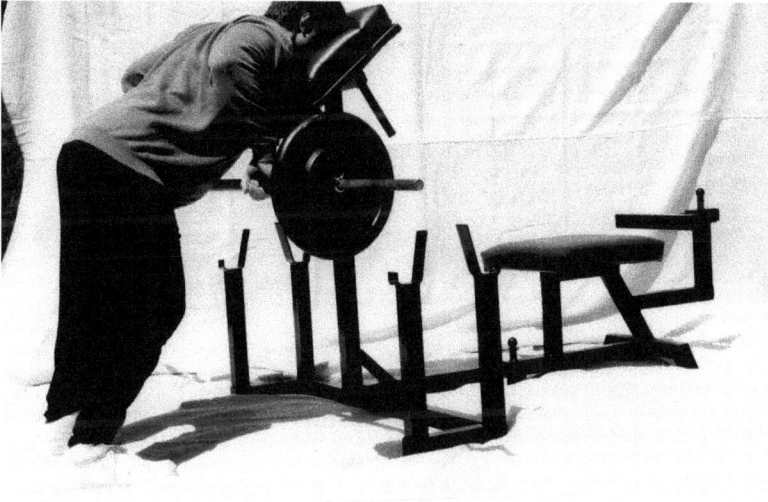

Appendix C

KC Row Bench Prototype

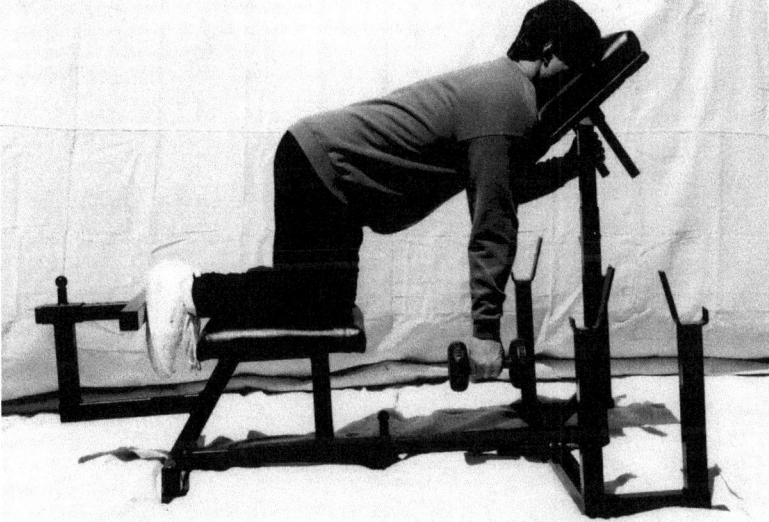

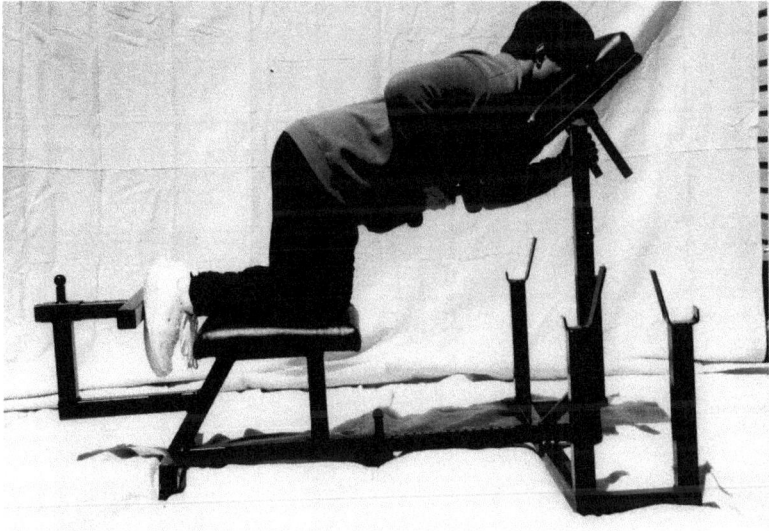

The Reach for the Ring

Notes

Notes

Notes

Notes

Notes